CHILD LABOUR REHABILITATION IN INDIA

HIMALAYAN RESEARCH AND CULTURAL FOUNDATION

The Himalayan Research and Cultural Foundation, an NGO in Special Consultative Status with ECOSOC, United Nations, is a multi-disciplinary research, cultural and development facilitative organisation engaged in appraising and creating awareness about various issues related to the Himalayan and trans-Himalayan regions in South and Central Asia, or parts thereof connected with its environment, biodiversity, regional development, human resources, history, culture, art and literature, social structures, economies, human rights, peace processes etc., thus contributing to sustainable development and promotion of human, educational and economic advancement of the peoples of the region, besides preserving and enriching their rich and variegated cultural heritage. The Foundation has evolved as a vibrant national centre specialised on the Hindu Kush-Himalayan and trans-Himalayan regions in South and Central Asia. By means of its publications and activities, the Foundation has been providing a specialised input and expert analysis on a wide range of issues.

OUR PUBLICATIONS

BOOKS

Afghanistan Factor in Central and South Asian Politics
Edited by K. Warikoo (New Delhi, 1994), 73 pp.

Society and Culture in the Himalayas
Edited by K. Warikoo (New Delhi, 1995), 316 pp.

Central Asia: Emerging New Order
Edited by K. Warikoo (New Delhi, 1995), 352 pp.

Jammu, Kashmir and Ladakh : Linguistic Predicament
Edited by P. N. Pushp and K. Warikoo (New Delhi, 1996), 224 pp.

Artisan of the Paradise: A Study of Art and Artisans of Kashmir
By D.N. Dhar (New Delhi: Bhavana Books & Prints, 1999), 230 pp.

Gujjars of Jammu and Kashmir
Edited by K. Warikoo (Bhopal, 2001), 317 pp.

Bamiyan: Challenge to World Heritage
Edited by K. Warikoo (New Delhi: Bhavana Books & Prints, 2002), xviii, 313pp. 61plates.

Mongolia-India Relations
By Oidov Nyamdavaa (New Delhi: Bhavana Books & Prints, 2003), 228pp.

JOURNAL

Himalayan and Central Asian Studies
(Quarterly being published regularly since 1997)

Child Labour Rehabilitation in India

Edited by

Bupinder Zutshi
Mondira Dutta

Issued under the auspices of

HIMALAYAN RESEARCH AND CULTURAL FOUNDATION
NEW DELHI

BHAVANA BOOKS & PRINTS
NEW DELHI

First Published 2003

ISBN 81-86505-64-4

Published by
BHAVANA BOOKS & PRINTS
101, AVG Bhawan, M-3, Connaught Circus,
New Delhi-110001 (India)
Phones: 011-23321198, 23415205 • Fax: 011-23415205
e-mail: rajanarya@vsnl.com

Printed by
ELEGANT PRINTERS
New Delhi-110064

Contents

Preface

Child labour particularly in hazardous industries has generated remarkable attention during the last one and a half-decades. This was due to the relentless efforts of the NGOs and other civil society organizations. Now it is being generally realized that, child labour especially in hazardous occupations is one of the worst social evils and has to be eliminated at the earliest. The Child Labour Act of 1986 and the Supreme Court directions of 1996 have made it imperative to withdraw children working in hazardous industries. It was felt that there was a need for a proper and holistic rehabilitation framework for the released children so that they may not re-enter into such occupations in future.

The book examines and evaluates the present educational and rehabilitation services provided by NGOs, Civil Society, Government agencies and UN agencies. The book has a collection of research papers, presented at the two-day international seminar on "Child Labour and their Rehabilitation: Some Issues". The workshop was organized by the Himalayan Research and Cultural Foundation (NGO in Special Consultative Status with ECOSOC, United Nations) in New Delhi on 30-31 July 1999. The seminar cum workshop was supported by International Labour Organization (New Delhi) and Association of Voluntary Action/ South Asian Coalition on Child Servitude (New Delhi).

The seminar cum workshop provided an excellent opportunity to have a direct interface between the academics, social scientists, government officials, international agencies, rehabilitation and funding agencies, social workers, NGOs, media persons, grass root level workers besides the children themselves who have been withdrawn from work. It was widely represented by National Human Rights Commission of India, Ministry of labour, Ministry of textiles (Government of India), various international organizations like; ILO, UNICEF, UNESCO, World Bank, UNDP, German Embassy, etc. Several rehabilitation agencies like; REHA (Consortium of Germany and India), RUGMARK, Terre des hommes, Save the Children (Canada), Centre for the Concern for Child Labour, Peace Trust, Project Mala, SACCS, Bachpan Bachhao Aandolan and Mukti Ashram participated in the workshop. Their contribution was significant in the formulation of recommendations. Field based NGOs from the carpet belt of Mirzapur - Bhadhoi, Bihar, M.P, Rajasthan, Tamil Nadu and Kashmir also participated in the workshop. Children released from hazardous industries also shared their concerns. Academicians from Jawaharlal Nehru University, Delhi University, Jamia Milia Islamia, National Council of Educational Research and Training, Institute of Public Opinion, Indian Social Institute, leading advocates of Supreme Court, Social activists and educational consultants attended the workshop. Representatives from Carpet Export Promotion Council and All India Carpet Manufacturers Association also participated in the seminar.

The book presents 19 research articles, covering components on child labour rehabilitation issues and examines the rehabilitation strategy undertaken by government, civil society and NGO sector in India. The articles provide a deep insight to the Child labour rehabilitation issues and strategies adopted for their eradication. The research articles are supported by substantial statistical information with a theoretical and conceptual understanding.

L. Mishra in his article "Child Labour: A Resume" presents several alarming facts about the child labour scenario in India. Major theme of his article is that "welfare is no substitute for freedom" and rehabilitation should be looking forward to the "indescribable joys of freedom." He states that, there will be a time when the children will mobilize and organize themselves and demand for their liberation from the shackles and fetters which have chained them for generations and robbed them of their basic rights unless they are given their due.

M.N. Venkatachaliah in his article "Child Labour Contemporary Realities" points out, that child labour is really a problem of lack of child education and lack of initiative on the part of the civil society to extract their due entitlements from the political society. He enumerates that these two are the most crucial links in a vicious circle and if unhooked, would usher empowerment of the civil society. The article not only presents statistical evidence of large-scale disparities in human development index between developed and under-developed countries but also presents large scale inter state disparities in human development index within the states in India. His article highlights the decay of the middle class and a rise of corruption at all levels, which has demoralized the society and has increased the mood of cynicism, resignation and abandonment among the society, in order to contain the social evils like child labour. The quintessence of his article is the universal education in order to break the concentration of wealth, status and power for a equitable distribution.

Kailash Satyarthi in his article questions the term 'rehabilitation of children' as being inappropriate, as majority of them have never been habilitated earlier. He believes that rehabilitation is a comprehensive process starting with identification, release, rehabilitation, as well as punishments to be meted out to the offenders. He states that there is a lack of compassion, spirit, and values while addressing the child labour issues. He believes that the whole issue of rehabilitation needs to be perceived as human rights' issue and not one of welfare.

C.J. Geogre in his article " Approaches Towards Combating Child Labour" examines the magnitude and causes of child labour in various economic activities. It also examines and provides suggestions for issues related to child labour amelioration, regulation, elimination, and eradication.

I.P. Massey in his article "Conceptual Narratives in Human Rights of the Child Discourse in Developing Countries" presents a historical perspective of various human rights conventions and constitutional narratives for protecting children from abuse.

Mondira Dutta examines the magnitude of child labour in India with a particular emphasis on the girl children. Her results are based on secondary sources of information, namely the Census of India and the National Sample Survey. An identification of the cause-effect relationships of magnitude of child labour with other social and economic parameters have been statistically analysed.

P.D. Mathews and R.M. Pal have emphasized the relevance of compulsory and universal primary education as a major methodology to eradicate the child labour in India. The authors have substantiated this view with worldwide experiences. The authors have aptly enunciated the role of political society and government for initiating compulsory and universal primary education.

P. Das Gupta in her article has examined the non-formal education intervention as a methodology for a focused target group in order to mainstream them into formal education at a later stage. The article examines features, tasks and challenges of non-formal education in India.

Ramakant Rai and Kuldeep Narain Maurya have examined the holistic picture of policy decisions taken for child labour rehabilitation in India. It also enumerates the difficulties faced by NGOs for the implementation of the decisions related to the release and rehabilitation of child labour. Case studies have been utilized in highlighting the child labour abuses committed by employers. The paper presents suggestions and recommendations for eradicating the *nuisance of* child labour.

Robin Garland and David Rangpal presents the initiatives undertaken by Project Mala Schools. The article discusses imparting quality education to the children released from carpet weaving activities of Mirzapur-Bhadhoi carpet weaving areas. It reveals how quality education has effectively reduced child labour in the carpet weaving activity.

R.K. Khurana enunciates the initiatives of International Programme on Elimination of Child Labour (IPEC) in India to provide education through Non-formal education to children released from hazardous activities. It also provides assessment of the IPEC programme examining its achievements, effectiveness, strengths and weaknesses.

Geeta Singh presents a background of Reha programmes in India and scrutinizes a detailed methodology for undertaking major activities under the Reha Programmes. The author also examines the impact of Reha programmes in reducing child labour in the hazardous activities.

Bal Adhikar Pariyojana examines experiences of child-responsive and community approaches as a methodology for alternative learning in carpet-weaving region. A detailed strategy for partnership with women's self-help groups, community level environment building and convergence with the education department has been elucidated in the article.

S. Sondhi, J.Paul Bhaskar and T.S. Chaddha have highlighted efforts made by Rugmak Foundation, Peace Trust and Carpet Export Promotion Council respectively for imparting education and other rehabilitation schemes for the children withdrawn from hazardous activities. They have also elucidated several positive impacts as a result of their intervention in the reduction of child labour in hazardous activities.

Helen R. Sekar has explained, critiqued and examined the rehabilitation programmes undertaken by government of India, Ministry of Labour under ILO-IPEC programme in major states of India to provide educational and other rehabilitation services to the children withdrawn from hazardous activities.

Bupinder Zutshi has presented a detailed assessment and evaluation of educational and other rehabilitation programmes undertaken by NGOs supported by voluntary and government organizations. The evaluation study examines the nature of services provided and quality of education provided by the NGOs in Mirzapur-Bhadhoi carpet weaving region.

Recommendations for the effective networking among the NGOs, Civil Societies, UN agencies and Government organizations in providing quality education and rehabilitation services, which were adopted after the deliberations in the workshop are stated in the appendix. These recommendations merit serious consideration and immediate implementation by all concerned agencies in the welfare of children.

We are grateful for the perspectives that we have received from all eminent writers, who have contributed in an insight to the prevailing child labour rehabilitation issues and strategies in all its dimensions. We are grateful to the South Asian Coalition on Child Servitude (SACCS), International Labour Organization, New Delhi, Ministry of Labour, Government of India and the Himalayan Research and Cultural Foundation for providing us all possible support, cooperation and guidance in sponsoring the workshop in Delhi where most of the articles were deliberated.

BUPINDER ZUTSHI
MONDIRA DUTTA

List of Contributors

Bupinder Zutshi, Jawaharlal Nehru University, New Delhi

C.J. George, Terre Des Hommes, Pune.

David Rangpal, Director, Project Mala Schools.

Geeta Singh, Coordinator, Indian Reha Secretariat.

Helen Sekar, V.V. Giri National Labour Institute, Noida.

I.P. Massey, LL.M. (Calif., Berkeley), Ph.D., Member, State Human Rights Commission,. Himachal Pradesh and Fellow, Indian Institute of Advanced Study, Rashtrapati Niwas, Shimla.

J. Paul Baskar, Chairman Peace Trust, Near Police Colony, Trichy Road, Dindigul - 624 005.

K.N. Maurya, Consultant, UPVHA.

Kailash Satyarthi, Chairperson, South Asian Coalition on Child Servitude.

L. Mishra, Ex-Secretary, Ministry of Labour, Government of India.

M.N. Venkatachliah, Ex-Chief Justice and Ex-Chairperson, National Human Rights Commission of India.

Mondira Dutta, Jawaharlal Nehru University, New Delhi

P.D. Mathews, S.J., Programme Director, Programme for Legal Aid, Indian Social Institute, New Delhi.

P. Das Gupta, National Open School, New Delhi.

R.K. Khurana, Program Officer, ILO, Delhi.

R.M. Pal, Indian Social Institute.

Ramakant Rai, UPVHA, Lucknow.

Robin Garland, Chairman, Project Mala, UK.

S. Sondhi, Ex-Executive Director, RUGMARK FOUNDATION.

T.S. Chadha, Secretary, Carpet Export Promotion Council.

1

Child Labour: A Resume

L. Mishra

India has approximately 375 million children under the age of 14 years as estimated by Census of India in the year 2001. Out of these 255 million children belong to the age group of 5-14 years. Every year 21 million children are being born, of which 8 million die and 13 million survive. Despite a number of programmes such as ICDS, mass immunisation including pulse polio programme and massive programmes for promoting nutrition of children through mid-day meals all over the country, the crude birth and death rate in various parts of India notably in Bihar, Madhya Pradesh, Uttar Pradesh and Rajasthan have not shown substantial declining trends. These States contribute directly and indirectly to large families, limiting access to human resource development (education and skill training), avenues of employment, and contributing to low wages and, therefore, necessitate engagement of children at work.

The Fifth Educational Survey has indicated that 119 million children have some form of access to both formal and non-formal education and about 100 million children have no access to formal or non-formal education. All of the 119 million children having some form of access to educational opportunity; do not remain in the school right up to Class V at the lower primary stage and Class VII up to the post primary stage. Many of them drop out or are pulled out or pushed out of the school system on account of variety of compulsions—social, economic and cultural. A reasonably high rate of enrolment backed by poor retention and high drop-out rates, results in colossal waste of human resources. This is too large a number and too precious to be wasted as it represents the most precious of all human resources. Childhood represents the most tender, most formative and most impressionable stage of human development. If children are deprived of the access to educational opportunity at the school going age, they would be forced to stay at home doing nothing but sitting idle, taking care of siblings and discharge of various household chores. There is also a possibility that they would come out of the threshold of household to engage themselves in agriculture and allied occupations of their parents or to engage themselves in various forms of wage employment. They may be doing so of their own accord or in volition of existing laws or on account of the compulsions resorted to by parents. If children in their school going age and in the most tender, formative and impressionable age of human development are sent away to the world of work, instead of being sent to the school, the petals of childhood would wither away without blossoming into the flower of manhood/womanhood and youth. In either of the contingencies child labour virtually becomes co-terminus with educational deprivation. This is a matter of great anxiety of concern and needs to be thought over, critically analyzed and introspect as to who was responsible for the unfortunate situation resulting in educational deprivation of a large number of children numbering over 100 million.

Majority of the children do not join the world of work on their own but are pushed to work. As they are pushed to work, they are subjected to long and arduous hours of work. They are made to work in extremely difficult conditions and interact with dangerous chemicals, which make them prone to irreparable damage in terms of their health, psyche and total development. Such an unfortunate situation is the outcome of deadly mindsets or ill-conceived notions of parents as well as employers. The parents believe that children can substantially contribute to the process of incremental income generation in the family with low income. This is a myth as studies have shown that children even in the most hazardous industries, occupations and processes do not earn more than Rs. 3 to Rs. 5 per day while they are subjected to hard and gruelling manual labour of 8-10 hours without payment of any overtime. Accidents do take place maiming or crippling children or killing them or causing temporary/permanent disablement but these are seldom reported, even the necessary compensation is not deposited in majority of cases. If a balance sheet were drawn in an objective and dispassionate manner showing the assets on the one hand and the liabilities on the other, it would be evident that while the gains are temporary and fragile, the losses in terms of the damage, which are caused, are considerable.

Employers prefer to engage children on account of situations, which are bargaining and beneficial to them, as they have fixed mindsets. Employers feel and believe that children are un-unionised and, therefore, will not engage them in trade disputes. Besides, they do not have the power to bargain either individually or collectively. These mindsets are framed as they feel that children cannot be unionised since they lack the capability to bargain individually or collectively. They are pliable or manoeuvrable and subjected to exploitation in the most callous and insensitive manner. Several employers advocate that children have nimble fingers and, therefore, are more productive than adults. This again is a myth, as it is nowhere established that children are more skilled or more productive than adults. Nimble fingers of children are meant for doing arithmetic, reading and writing and not for engaging children in hard manual labour in hazardous occupations, industries and processes.

Such mindsets can only be removed with the help of a massive social mobilisation through involvement of anyone and everyone who has the right urge, inclination and commitment to work for elimination of child labour. What is more important in this process of social mobilisation is the ethos and spirit and not tons and tons of money. The desirable need is to bring together a confluence of creative forces and energies under umbrella of one association of creative thinkers, writers, artistes as had happened in the case of Total Literacy Campaign. This was not utopian but possible, feasible and achievable. Only through such a strategy and methodology social mobilisation could become a reality. Welfare was not a substitute for freedom as it represents the indescribable joy and purify of mind. If individuals and the society as a whole remain callous and insensitive about elimination of child labour, a day will come, when children will themselves mobilise and organise and demand their liberation from the shackles and fetters which have chained them for generations and robbed them of their basic rights. True rehabilitation could be meaningful when it was accompanied by the indescribable joy of freedom.

The central message in this entire campaign for mass mobilisation or social mobilisation should be the following:

- Childhood represents the most tender, formative impressionable stage of human development.
- Childhood is a stage of excitement and joy and access of education and is not the age for entering the world of work, which requires physical energy, mental and emotional maturity and psychological adaptability.
- Even if a child has been subejcted to the world of work and had lost the excitement and joy of childhood, everything is not lost and a working child can be released from work and rehabilitated through education which is the most important tool of liberation and reorganisation of a boy's and girl's life.
- This cannot evidently be the programme of one Ministry, one organisation or one agency and must be a global and national and collective concern.
- A model can be worked out exclusively the way the Total Literacy Campaign was worked out with Bharat Gyan Vigyan Samiti playing a catalytic role and government playing the promotional role to promote and facilitate creation of a climate or environment where elimination of child labour becomes a reality.

2

Child Labour: Contemporary Realities

M.N. Venkatachaliah

Child Labour eradication is a highly sensitive and a live issue as, 40% of our population consists of children below the age of 14 years, of them about 110 million are in the age group of 6 to 10 years. The total child population in India under the age of 14 years in itself is the sum total of the population of a number of countries. Their education is the biggest challenge. Some 67 million are supposed to have facilities for elementary education. But the quality is not uniform and sometimes borders on the dismal. 50% of the world's Leprosy afflicted, 40% of the world's Tuberculosis and 25% of the world's blind are in India. There is an immediate and dangerous prospect of the break-out in epidemic proportions of Malaria, Tuberculosis, Hepatitis and HIV and the Society is wholly unprepared for these challenges. Our inability to handle the forces of change is historic and proverbial.

Child labour is really the problem linked to lack of child education. These two are perhaps, the most crucial links in a vicious circle. If they were unhooked, the vicious circle would end ushering in the empowerment of the civil society. In India, contrary to the other developed countries, the civil society is unable to extract its due and entitlement from the political society. The civil society unfortunately is a heterogeneous agglomeration of groups, which are in constant conflict with each other. This non-coherence of the civil society was the cause for its lack of empowerment. Education of women and children is a significant contributing factor to a solution for several problems. Lack of education of the girl child is perhaps the key to most excruciating problems of the country. Several glaring disparities in the access to education, access to medical services, public distribution system between two states within India itself are witnessed. These disparities are as a result of lack of compulsory education.

Contemporary Realities: India's Social and Economic Infrastructure

The grandeur of Indian civilization and its great contribution to art, architecture and sculpture, its fascinating exposition of the concept of mind, time and consciousness, which can only be characterised as reflecting the peak of intellectual glory of the world, all seem today unreal in the context of the contemporary moral and social morass. Instances of bureaucratic aloofness and indifference, insolence of authority and power is the schism, between the political and the civil societies. A small man when clothed with authority unleashes a severe kind of tyranny and works in a determined manner to make the lives of his fellowmen miserable. India's problems today stem from venality of administration and insincerity and irreverence towards values. A commentator describing the political scene in America after the death of Abraham Lincoln said, "The age of heroes is gone. The scene is peopled with charlatans, quick-buck artistes and from muddled mediocre to the dangerously deranged". India has created for itself; by it own indiscipline, lethargy and corruption, immense economic and social problems. Indeed some of them might soon become insurmountable if they are not tackled and remedied immediately. It's amazing how the community in authority can do this to themself(ves). This is a suicidal, unilateral, voluntary educational disarmament of the country. As a community, we have been so insensitized and dehumanized by our pre-occupations with worldly goods, that nothing seems to ring in our minds. We have been so insensitive to one of the most crucial issues to the human rights dialogue of the country. Mere existence of endless number of phrases hardly has any matching performance in terms of action. It is high time that some systematic development of packages or programmes, which are economically viable, replicable and durable, be designed.

Great changes in technology will confront Indian industry with very severe challenges. The pace of change in the immediate five years is going to out-class the changes of the last hundred years. The perplexing inequities and crudities of the international economic order will aggravate India's economic vulnerabilities. India's economy is weak, fragile and vulnerable. Its GDP is just about one-third of a day's transactions on the New York Stock exchange. Indeed, according to 1998 Human Development report, the three richest persons in the world have assets that exceed the combined GDP of 48 least developed countries; the fifteen richest have assets that exceed the total GDP of sub-Saharan-Africa; the wealth of thirty-two richest persons exceeds the total GDP of South-Asia; the assets of eighty-four richest exceed the GDP of China with 1.2 billion population. Of 4.4 billion people in developing countries, nearly 60% (uniformity) live without basic sanitation, **one-third** without safe drinking water, **one-fourth** without adequate housing, **one-fifth** do not study beyond grade 5 and **one-fifth** are severely under- nourished. The same report estimates that the additional cost for achieving and maintaining universal access to basic education for all, basic health for all, reproductive health care for all women, adequate food for all, safe water and sanitation for all, is roughly Rs 40 billion a year less than 4% of the combined wealth of the 225 richest persons of the world. Their assets when added, equal those of 47% of the world's population (2.5 billion people).

In 1750, India's share of world's manufacturing output was 24.5%, while that of Japan 3.8%, U.K. 1.9% and USA 0.1%. Today India's share in the global GDP is 0.9%. In just 10 years of the nineteen eighties the expenditure of Governments, Central and States increased from 11.8% of the GDP to 23%. In the last few years of this decade the Central Governments' expenditure rose from Rs.92, 808 crore to a staggering Rs.2, 68,107 crores. The deficit in 1948-49 budget was Rs. 1 crore. In 1997-98 it become Rs.86, 345 crores.

India, Uttar Pradesh and Kerala: Contrasts in Access to Public Services

	India	*Uttar Pradesh*	*Kerala*
Percentage of rural children aged 12-14 who have never been enrolled in a School, 1986-87			
Female	51	68	1.8
Male	26	27	0.4
Proportion of children aged 1-13 months Who have not received any vaccination, 1992-93(%)	30	43	11
Percentage of recent births preceded by Antenatal check up, (1992-93)	49	30	97
Proportion of births taking place in medical Institutions, 1991 (%)	24	4	92
No. of hospital beds per million persons 1991	732	340	2,418
Proportion of villages with medical facilities	14	10	96
Proportion of the population receiving subsidized cereals from the public Distribution system (1986-87) (%)	29	3	87

Decay of the Middle Class and Corruption

Here again we have an uncontrolled epidemic of corruption in public life. Mechanisms to stem the rot have proved futile. Disenchantment with legal processes has demoralised the society. There is an increasing mood of cynicism, resignation and abandonment. The great Indian middle class who was a cultural bastion has all but disappeared. There is an imminent collapse of the political system and conditions of near anarchy. The well-to-do will soon seek to live in private fortresses protected by private armies. Their children will go to school and play under the surveillance of armed guards.

Pawan Varma, in his book, 'The great Indian middle class', refers to the critical implications of corruption on social sentience:

> "Corruption at the highest levels was now assumed to be the norm. Its existence was taken for granted. Allegations sprouted quick and fast from what was undoubtedly a fertile field of evidence. Suspicions matured overnight into beliefs, and beliefs, in turn, nurtured new suspicions."

The man in the street says to himself: Well if everybody seems corrupt, why shouldn't I be corrupt? . . . This new reality dictated that honesty was the flip side of the coin of failure, and dishonesty was the unavoidable accompaniment of success. The successful were there for all to see. And as their number audaciously proliferated, the wall of reticence and inhibition against the means they had adopted began to crumble. The belief that corruption was rampant prepared the ground for it to grow further, casting a shadow on almost every aspect of the nation's life. And the perception that it was pervasive, legitimised its existence.

Corruption of this nature had existed even before, but the scale and blatancy with which it now seemed to be entrenched was something new. As the victim of this escalation, the average middle-class person was a vehement critic of corruption. But in the general erosion of ethics, many of the newly corrupt were people from his own class.

In its ambitions for upward movement, the middle class lost its sensitivity to suffering and poverty and became acutely acquisitive. Tolerance of corruption and immorality and gradual acquiescence in them are inevitable consequences. An industrialist estimates that three items alone, i.e. the losses from substandard quality of civil contracts, crop-loss owing to defective systems of storage and theft of electricity, amounts to something like Rs.50,000 crores annually. A professor said: India is today trapped into a state of growing anarchy. Events are overtaking us with rapidity, which is bewildering. Leaders are not in command of the situation with actions having unintended effects. The growing conflict, lack of credibility of leaders and institutions, decline of institutions and fragmentation of society has led to this state of affairs. Energies are getting dissipated in fire-fighting rather than in building a thought through future.

One of the ills of Indian society was that those who were possessed of wealth and those who were leaned did not even think it was possible that the small man would, one day, assert his place under the Sun.

At such critical times a tendency to decry democracy and its institutions becomes fashionable. Some tend to blame our political institutions and say that we have too much democracy and that it is not good. The choice, they say, is between good-governance and too much of self-governance. This argument is again a red herring. As pointed by a professor: "The arguments that India's problems are a result of too much democracy and/or high population growth are invalid. Underlying these arguments is an elitist notion, which is the real source of the problem since it undermines democracy. The issue surely is, too much power in a few who misused it and made the citizen helpless and a cynic. The remedy is not more freedom of action of a few or for insulating them from popular pressures in the shape of either a national or a presidential form of government, but to make the rulers subject to the scrutiny of the citizen, to curb the excesses of the few."

> "*Seek Ye First The* Kingdom of Politics
> *All Else Will Be Added* Unto You."

These words were etched in stone at the base of the statue of Dr. Nkrumah outside the law courts in Accra. They shocked the world, but one increasingly realises that they exposed the true face of political realities. When political climate and political processes become impure, it is unrealistic to be astonished, if there is no decorous deference to the rules of the constitutional game. Rule of law, democracy and the fundamental organisations of a self-governing people are all reduced to a farce. Disillusionment kills ideas and promotes forces of defilement of institutions: a sure precursor of anarchy.

Electoral system and practices have been the ugly sources of corruption. Britain got over its enormous problems by a meticulous analysis of the sources of corruption and establishment of institutions of good governance. A scientific approach to the problems of government was adopted laying them open to the scrutiny of investigation, of exact knowledge, of statistical information and to a ruthless pursuit of the utilitarian doctrine of the greatest good of the greatest number. The consequences, in administrative terms, were economy, efficiency, inspection and control. The sources of corruption indeed are the concentration of 'power', 'wealth' and 'status' in one individual or a group of individuals collectively. Prime Minister John Major's recent Citizens' Charters have made significant contribution to good governance.

Education: Source of Empowerment of Civil Society

One of the means of breaking the concentration of wealth, status and power—a deadly combination in which corruption thrives—is empowerment of the civil society. Education, particularly of women, has demonstrated its great potential in empowering the civil society to extract its entitlements from the political society. Dr.Amartya Sen and Jean Dreze illustrate the difference in social opportunity that female literacy has brought about in Kerala in their studies.

The greatest harm of this increasing cynicism about standards in public life and instability of social order has brought about the disruption of family values. The immensity of the harm that the collapse of family values will bring in, is not sufficiently realized, even as the extent and gravity of the damage already done and its implications are not fully grasped.

3

Child Labour Issues and Rehabilitation—A Thematic Presentation

Kailash Satyarthi

Background

In the last decade the issue of child labour has sprung on top of the national agenda in India and many other countries. Due to the relentless efforts of the NGOs and other social development organisations it has been realised that child labour is one of the worst social evils and has to be eliminated at the earliest. This can only be achieved with a concrete time bound strategy and action plan of which *rehabilitation* is an integral part.

Concept

The ambit of rehabilitation is vast and at this point it would be pertinent to have a clear understanding on what all it encompasses. There can be various interpretations of this term but unfortunately the general perception of it is quite limited, which sometimes proves to be counter productive for the overall development of a child.

Rehabilitation vs Habilitation

When we talk of rehabilitation, we assume that the children freed from labour need support for being reintegrated into the social mainstream. But the pertinent question is, whether the word 'rehabilitation' is appropriate, in relation to most cases of child labour. The fact is that these children don't even have proper 'habilitation'. On the contrary its conspicuous absence in backward areas and communities push the poverty strucked illiterate families to give in to the basic demands of existence and accept the brutal terms of the employers and their agents by sending their tender aged children to work. It needs to be probed whether we are providing them with facilities of education, vocational training, housing, and employment etc. or reassuring them about what they have in the past.

We can enumerate this with an example. In the month of July SACCS rescued 26 children from the carpet industries of Allahabad. After the completion of basic bureaucratic formalities they were taken back to their hometown in Saharsa (Bihar). An activist accompanying them called me that he has not been able to trace their families. They had no homes. Everything had been washed away by the perennial floods of Bihar and the families had got scattered—some sitting on treetops, some had gone to higher lands and some were lost. It was a dilemma for the activists on how to rehabilitate the children under such circumstances. The point being made is that when we have not been able to provide secure housing, employment etc to the people in all these years, is it not quite offbeat to talk about rehabilitation ?

A Project or a Process

Today rehabilitation is becoming restricted to a project or a programme. A defined mechanical programme is run and we feel satisfied of having rehabilitated a fixed number of children in a stipulated time frame and fund-oriented framework. It may sound cynical but the Indian politicians have reduced living human beings with flesh and blood to mere ballots and votes—as Hindu, Muslim, Sikh, dalits, brahamans, etc. Unfortunately, the NGO sector have reduced our children to a fixed number of faceless beneficiaries. If an NGO has a programme for rehabilitation of 35 children it feels satisfied after having achieved that goal, but perhaps another child at the doorstep of the rehabilitation centre who probably needs rehabilitation much more, goes unnoticed. Society's responsibility to rehabilitate these children is no less than the rest. Therefore, rehabilitation has to be evolved as a value and wholesome process.

Child Welfare or Child Right

Many times attitude, not only of the bureaucrats, who run the rehabilitation process after rescue of the children, but also of the rehabilitating NGOs, is that of charity. The recipients of the benefits, out of ignorance, have a feeling of being obliged. The financial aids or other benefits reach the children after lengthy red-tapism and harassment of the parents and the children. There has to be a change in this attitude. Rehabilitation process is a child's right and not an obligation. This requires a good amount of effort of continuous awareness building in the community including the parents and a systematic orientation of officials and social workers.

A Government or an NGO Responsibility

There has been a lack of clarity on whether rehabilitation process is the sole responsibility of the government or of the NGOs and other social organisations. The government is and should be the absolute capable institution to handle the process of rehabilitation. It is not possible by NGOs to rehabilitate the 60 million child labourers in the country. NGOs can most certainly work as catalysts and set precedents or models for the government to replicate and if necessary improve upon them as policies. NGOs can work in co-ordination with the administration but the ultimate onus lies with the government.

Material or Emotional

Rehabilitation, as understood by most of us, is material convalescence. The children are given financial aids or other benefits under the rehabilitation programmes. But this is not sufficient. Many times the children are so traumatised that they need much more than just material things. Rehabilitation demands emotional support. Children are unable to bare the tortures and exploitation of the employers and become disoriented and highly insecured. They need counselling and reassurance that they are safe. It is a sad reality that no one can retrieve the child labourers their most valued things in life—their childhood and their precious time. But we can make all efforts to make them realise that they are free and normal human beings. They have rights and opportunities and there are people to take care of them and protect their rights. Further more efforts must be made to reinforce their hopes, aspirations and their dreams during the course of rehabilitation.

I quote an example from my personal experience during the Global March Against Child Labour held last year across 133 countries. A 13-year-old Cambodian girl Pao was marching with us as a core marcher. She was a former child labour who had been sold thrice, once as a child domestic, then in a brothel and finally in a nightclub, before being rescued by some local NGOs. I observed that she remained aloof unlike others shouting and playing child core marchers. Then one day finding me alone she came up to me and asked me, " Tell me am I still a child?" This was the first time I had heard her talk ever since the March had begun. I pulled her close to me and assured her that she was very much a child and that she had all the rights to enjoy her childhood just as the others did. She wept for more than an hour clinging on me and I kept reassuring and consoling her. The next morning we were all very surprised to see that Pao was amongst the leaders shouting the slogans and walking hand in hand with the other marchers.

On another occasion in the SACCS run Mukti Ashram, there were great celebration when one of the rescued boys from the carpet industry, Nageshwar got back his voice after weeks of loss of speech due to the trauma he had suffered. He was confined in a small one-room workplace with 6 other fellow child slaves for 7 years. When he attempted to escape, he was branded with hot iron rods all over the body and thus he lost his speech.

Rehabilitation—A Standard Format

All child labourers are brought under the purview of the same rehabilitation programmes irrespective of the nature of the situational environment of the rescued child labour. Children freed from carpet looms or similar places are dealt under the same rehabilitation programmes as those working as part time child labourers. These children have psychological, mental and physical health problems. Children from the carpet industry suffer from serious breathing ailments and children of the glass industry often suffer from T.B. A mere compensation in terms of money is not sufficient to the parents, as it does not suffice the requirements of the child. The children cannot be rehabilitated with a standard format of education, training or financing. It should be designed depending on the circumstances and condition of the child rescued.

Rehabilitation—Main Stream Education vs. Non-Formal Education

Nowadays, the government or non-governmental rehabilitation programmes for the children generally focus on non-formal education. It seems that the safest and the easiest intervention, is that of 'NFE centres'. But it has been observed that the programme engages the children only for 2-3 hours a day. This gives them ample scope to get back to child labour in factories or other work places. Moreover, this sort of education demarcates the child from the other children of the society. It gives rise to a feeling of inequality amongst the children, which should be discouraged. Programmes should be oriented towards mainstream education, which would also work as a catalyst to bring the children at par with the other children.

The Constraints

It is unfortunate that rehabilitation has remained a grey area despite so many efforts to eradicate child labour. In fact, SACCS, which has the credit of rescuing more than 50,000 child labourers over the past two decades, observes that the area of rehabilitation has been ignored the most. There have been only a few rehabilitation programmes that have shown tangible results like that of M.V. Foundation, the SACCS run ashrams.

Government—Apathy

As mentioned earlier, the major responsibility of rehabilitation lies on the government but it has failed to effectively work on those lines. The existing government schemes on rehabilitation of child labour/ bonded child labour are incomprehensive and obsolete as they were designed in the late 70's (twenty years ago) and that too for bonded labour in general and not particularly for bonded child labourers.

The National Child Labour Project (NCLP) scheme of the

government is equally outdated and as such has not yielded any satisfactory results due to in-built lacunae and poor implementation policies. For example, the beneficiary children under these schemes are not actual child labourers for whom the funds were mainly allocated. Though the programme was successful in Saharsa (Bihar), Virudhnagar (T.N.), Mandsaur (M.P.) and a few other places and could be run as model schools but due to the lax attitude of the government it could not be followed up.

The Supreme Court ruling of December 10, 1996 has been in vain as under this ruling, there is no scheme to evolve funds for education or rehabilitation for child labour. The scheme stipulates that an amount of Rs. 20,000 is to be collected as fine from the employer and Rs. 5000 to be given by the government in each case of child employment. This is so because there are very few cases of actual implementation of this ruling.

Under the present scheme of centrally sponsored relief for rehabilitation of freed child bonded labourers, officially released children and the parents of freed bonded child labourers are entitled to get earning assets like milk cattle, bullock cart, small shops, poultry farms, rickshaws etc. amounting to Rs. 10,000. Also under other existing schemes, if child labourers are SC/ST or below the poverty line, children below 14 are to be sent to schools and their families entitled to facilities like land and housing. Unfortunately, this scheme can never be implemented successfully due to the absence of rigorous follow-up action.

Delay in implementation and corruption

There is no co-ordination in between release and rehabilitation. There are cases when the rescued child labourer has to wait for years before getting any benefits of rehabilitation. Even the ex-gratia which is meant to be given on the spot at the time of rescue is not given. This frustrates the parents and the children so much so that it in fact acts as a causative for them to go back to the same situation of servitude.

Tremendous corruption is encountered in every steps. One such incident of gross corruption and lack in foresight some years ago in Mirzapur occurred when around 200 child labourers had been rescued from the carpet belt of Mirzapur-U.P. and were officially rehabilitated in a cluster of villages. When spoken to the children and their families, it was found that each one of them had been given mercifully a pair of undergarments and receipt on which they were made to put their thumb impressions, shockingly recorded that they have been given garment shops by the government. Even if one ignores the corruption, who can justify opening of over 20 garment shops in a very poor village of 300 inhabitants? After a rigorous effort by SACCS in this matter an inquiry was set–up by the government and some of the officials were transferred.

Moreover, the allocated funds do not reach the right quarters in most cases. It was found that funds allocated for schools are not spent in the right manner. For e.g. since the last six months the NCLP run schools are finding it hard to run due to scarcity of funds in the Saharsa district of Bihar. On being asked the officials justify that an inquiry commission has been set-up to find out the reasons for the closure of schools. Meanwhile, the children are being victimised due to this government fallout.

Lack of Conceptual Clarity on Child Labour

There is a fundamental ideological or conceptual difference amongst NGOs regarding elimination of child labour. There are many NGOs and government officials who run rehabilitation programmes with an understanding that rehabilitation could go hand in hand with regularised child labour. Many of them feel that after completion of rehabilitation project the children can find better jobs with improvised wages, working and living conditions. This is a counter productive approach. The complete elimination of child labour has to be the singular goal in mind when the rehabilitation process is designed and implemented.

Conclusion

First of all, the child labour prone areas as well as child labour catchments areas have to be identified carefully. The government should initiate comprehensive development programme for the habilitation in those areas including proper land reforms, housing under several government schemes, income generation activities focussing women in the community, employment opportunities, easy banking and credit facilities, irrigation, minimum wage etc. To stop the engagement of children in the labour market, it is essential for the government to implement various poverty alleviation programmes on priority basis in such areas. The government, on top priority, must ensure free, compulsory and meaningful basic education for all the children up to the age of fourteen.

A National Commission on Child Labour/Servitude should be constituted at the earliest. Such a commission should not entrusted only with the task of investigation or inquiry, but it should have executive powers to implement the programme of identification, rescue and rehabilitation of child labourers. The commission will carry out rehabilitation through NGOs, government departments, UN agencies etc. and monitor the same. Such a commission should also be empowered to initiate litigation against the offenders before the competent judicial institutions. This should be comprised of a sitting or former judge of the Supreme Court; eminent social activists involved in the issue of child labour, government bureaucrats with proven record in social field and other members from the judiciary.

Until such a commission is formed, the National Human Rights Commission should be entrusted to set up a sub-commission/committee with all the authorities and adequate budgets and manpower to perform the aforesaid task.

Rehabilitation should be a process of reintegration of the children with the society in every aspect. Due to isolation and exploitation the children get unaccustomed to the society and are unable to mix with them. The rehabilitation programmes should be able to orient them to place themselves as respectable members of the society. The families and in a broader term the society should also be oriented to accept the children back.

The Rehabilitation programmes should be child centered. When such a rehabilitation programme is designed, inputs from the parents as well as the children should be taken into account. Rehabilitation of the child should be in a holistic manner. It should cater to his psychological, mental, physical, educational, emotional and sociological needs.

As mentioned above in this paper, there is no state sponsored comprehensive policy strategy, scheme or action plan for the rehabilitation of released child labourers. Up till now, two very obsolete and failed schemes i.e. centrally sponsored scheme for rehabilitation of bonded labourers and national child labour project are in common practice. Hence, there is an urgent need of designing such a holistic time bound applicable scheme, which must be monitored at various levels. An adequate budgetary allocation should also be made.

A proper orientation and training should be given to all those governmental and non-governmental institutions and personnels that are engaged in the rehabilitation of child labourers.

4

Approaches Towards Combating Child Labour

C. J. George, Terre Des Hommes

Child Labour: Violation of Children's Rights

A child employed is a future denied; a future denied for itself and for society. Child labour amounts to violation of children's rights in total, right to survival with dignity, right to develop and right to be protected from exploitation of all kinds. Large numbers of children employed, is a denial of the future for the nation and for the world. It amounts to utter wastage of human potentials. Employment of children, which is the hallmark of poverty, underdevelopment, illiteracy, deprivation, uneven development, concentration of wealth and resources, etc., becomes ultimately also, a cause of all these maladies. The vicious circle of exploitation, deprivation and domination and subjugation thus gets perpetuated.

Magnitude of the Problem

The fact however today is that, at least 120 million children between the ages of 5-14 years are employed full time all over the world. (Estimate of ILO's Bureau of Statistics). A vast majority of these are in the developing continents of Asia, Africa and Latin America. It is also estimated that an equal number of children, if not more, are part time employed or are part of the marginal work force.

Estimation of the magnitude of child labour has always been difficult for a variety of reasons. There is no single definition of child labour. There are also different positions on what constitutes 'a child'. Children are found employed by different sections of employers but they also work along with their family at home and outside. Sometimes they are working while attending school and have some leisure but often they are engaged full time. Sometimes they assist parents who are working for others like in the case of beedi-rolling, brick kilns, etc., but at other times they are helping them in household activities or on their own farms. Children are also found self employed, for instance street children. Sometimes they are also entrepreneurs. There are cases where children are not doing any productive work or rendering any service but are earning an income as is the case in those who indulge in begging. Here again they are often employed in begging by adults. Thus the whole scenario is very complex. Also there are instances (e.g. children engaged in prostitution to earn a livelihood) where the nature of services may not constitute labour but are definitely exploitative. The comprehensive definition of child labour which reads "Child labour includes children prematurely leading adult lives, working with or without wages; under conditions damaging to their physical, mental, social, emotional and spiritual development, denying them their basic rights to education, health and development" is compiled on the basis of the effect on the child and not on the basis of employee-employer relationship or generation of assets or rendering of services

There are also arguments that in the case of children below the compulsory schooling age; all children out of schools must be considered as child labour. For instance in India all children between 6 to 14 years of age who are out of school should be considered as child labour.

Sectors of Employment

The sectors in which children are found working are also numerous. They are found in many sectors of agriculture, manufacturing and services. They are also labouring in ancillary sectors, fish farming, stone quarries, mining, animal husbandry, horticulture, trade, factories, service sectors like hotels, garages cleaning sewage clearance, vending, deep sea fishing, beedis, fire works, matches, bangles, rag picking, and numerous other sectors. Large numbers of children work in occupations and processes, which are inherently hazardous. This apart, any form of labour, hazardous or otherwise, performed for a long period of time without adequate leisure and rest become hazardous for the young bodies and minds, retarding their growth and development. Hence viewed this from the child's position, all forms of employment at least up to a certain age are hazardous.

Rate of Participation in Labour

There are considerable differences in the incidence of child labour among continents and nations. For instance, while India has the largest number of child labour and children out of school, the rate of participation of children in the total labour force is lower than other countries. According to ILO estimates 61% of the 250 million odd children in the age group of 5-14 who are employed can be found in Asia, 3.1% in Africa and 0.7 % in Latin America. If India is considered as an example, 12.7 million are full time employed 10.5 million part time labourers or (marginal labourers) and the ones who are out of school may be about 60 million. But this large number accounts only for 5.2 % of the total labour force, where as the share of child labour within the total in other countries is:

- 27.3% in Turkey
- 20.7 % in Thailand
- 19.5 % in Bangladesh
- 16.6 % in Pakistan
- 12.4 % in Indonesia
- 11.5 % in Mexico
- 8.2 % in Egypt
- 4.4 % in Sri Lanka
- 18.8 % in Brazil

Causes

Child labour is a structural phenomenon. The unjust, in egalitarian, exploitative, socio-economic, political structure, which breeds poverty and deprivation, generates child labour too. While poverty is certainly a contributive factor it cannot be viewed in isolation. The exploitative structures which cause deprivations create the need for children to seek early employment in order to contribute to their and the families survival, also create a demand for cheap labour compounded by unemployment and under employment. Thus the causes of child labour cannot be isolated from the structural dynamics, which create and perpetuate the state of poverty, exploitation and marginalisation. Control over natural resources and productive assets by a small section of the population globally, nationally and locally, remain at the center of the causative factors of this social and economic evil too.

Possible Remedies

Logically the remedies to any phenomenon should relate to its causes. Remedies that do not do so give temporary relief or superficial treatment. So if it is agreed that the causes leading to employment of a large number of children are structural, then all efforts to alter this situation must address the causal factors. Only structural changes which promote fair adult wages, adult employment, access to natural resources and means of production like land, water, social integration and justice, gender equity, universal access to relevant education, etc., can create the ground for ending child labour as a practice. These structural changes may take place either through a revolutionary change or an evolutionary process. The latter disrupts the prevalent social and productive relations totally and ushers, in new forms of social relations or productive relations. The old structures are revamped and new social structures created. However, the new structures may ensure the absence of child labour only, in as far as, the commitment of the revolutionary forces to such values.

The evolutionary form of social change, bringing in the guarantee for the rights of the children, women and other marginalised groups is more common place currently. Such efforts stem from the concerted actions on different elements of the structures, though not at once, but with coordination. While the points of activity are specific, they are not viewed in isolation but are expected to compliment each other. Such attempts bring in gradual change in the situation.

Debates on Child Labour

Child labour is widely discussed today. Debates on whether child labour is a result of poverty or a cause of poverty are currently prevalent. While social scientists and political activists emphasizing delineate the structural causes that only structural change can ensure the end of this practice, the philanthropists argue that it is better to light one candle rather than grope through darkness and analyse the reasons. There are also those who prescribe a one-point programme of free compulsory education for eradication of child labour. The poverty argument itself is viewed by many as an 'alibi' and excuse to justify and perpetuate the practice. Corresponding to different positions there are also different approaches to combat the problem of child labour.

Prevalent Approaches

Analysis, understanding or logic is not always the starting point of social intervention. Very often such interventions are a spontaneous response to concrete situation witnessed at a point of time. The response often could be so spontaneous as to make it simplistic. This also may be confined only to a particular instance or situation without even recognizing the fact that the instance in consideration is one among the numerous such instances in the society.

Responses also often follow the social position of the people concerned and their own understanding of the social problems. Child labour has come to attract the attention of a large number of people, groups, political parties, labour unions, national governments, international organisations from development and human rights concerns, employer's and NGO's of national and international coverage. This has resulted in a large pool of approaches and methodologies being considered and affected towards tackling the situations of child labour. While most of these approaches are complementary to each other, others are not so. This has also led to a wide debate among different sections of people on strategies for dealing with the practice of child labour. It is expected that the debate is often coloured by the social and political positions and assumptions of the involved parties. The approaches and positions are as diverse, if not more, as the problem itself is.

Producer and Product Focussed Strategies

Traditionally most efforts to combat child labour started with the child labourers. But new initiatives have some times adopted the products or the markets as the starting point. The all-pervasive influence of the market and trade relations, which are specific to the present era, is attempted to be tapped through such approaches. Thus the current measures taken against child labour can basically be grouped under child labour (producer) focussed and the product/market focussed ones.

Child Labour Focussed Approaches

Child Labourer Amelioration

Amelioration of the existential suffering of the labouring child is the concern of such an approach. The approach may be motivated by a sense of pity, charity or kindness towards the child concerned. This approach is more individually focussed and does not necessarily consider the situation of a large number of children having to work in adverse conditions.

The 'child must be helped' constitutes the attitude. There are not many questions asked or causes sought after. Long term solutions for the individual child or group of children may or may not be considered. However the urgency is to immediately help the child or children concerned personally. The kind of assistance provided by such approach could be varied. It could be to help the child with some additional facilities while continuing to work or it could also be to remove them from working situations and provide an alternative.

Individual attention care and a personalized interest would be the main stay of this approach. Such approaches are not only adopted by individuals but even by organisations. A relationship of patronage is often a hallmark of this approach. The assistance offered to the child and the kindness extended might include the family of the child but normally would not go beyond that.

The approach is a personalized and supports individual child. But does not amount to be a social intervention as no efforts to tackle the social problem are included. The approach could lead to paternalistic and dependency relationship.

Child Labour Regulation

The child labour regulation approach has various shades and positions within itself. The approach starts from a position that child labour is a fact of life. There is no easy solution for it. This is a necessary evil. Poverty and social structures are responsible for it. You cannot change the situation where by the children do not have to work. If children are taken out of work, their families and they themselves will suffer irreparable losses. Their survival itself will be a problem.

Children are working because there is a need to work. Their earnings are crucial for them and the families' existence. But they are being exploited in the process. They have to work very long hours. They work for low wages. They do not have the possibility to attend school. They lack leisure and rest. They lack medical care and attention. They work in difficult situations and so on. However, taking them out of the working situation is not a practical solution.

Consequently the solution to the suffering and deprivation of the labouring children is found in measures, which will regulate their work, the working conditions, wages, period of work, etc. The regulation is done both by invoking employers and also by seeking legal intervention by the Government. Demands are made to reduce working hours, to allow rest period at regular intervals, to provide educational and medical care to working children and to pay them fair wages. It is hoped that an acceptable condition of labour can be obtained by introducing appropriate conditions.

Certain regulations tend to see child labour as a permanent phenomenon, while others view it as a practical need at present, as elimination or abolition is not feasible. Consequently they would argue for the rights of child labourer as in the case of 'labourer'. Right to organize trade unions, fair minimum wages, right to participate, etc. is demanded for the toiling children. It is also argued sometimes that as the situation necessitates the entry of children into labour, no minimum age of entry to child labour shall be enforced. A child must have the right to work if situation so demands. It is further emphasized that the child should have the 'right to work with dignity'.

It is often forgotten that children are employed primarily because they constitute cheap labour. If all these kinds of regulations have to be imposed, there may be no reason left to employ children.

Yet another position stands for regulating employment of children in some sectors while prohibiting it in other sectors. The sectors in which children are found employed are divided into hazardous sectors and non-hazardous sectors. For instance, the legislation in India prohibits the employment of children below 14 years of age in hazardous industries and seeks to regulate the same in non-hazardous sectors. Hazardous or not is decided according to nature of operations or conditions of work. In other words only those processes of work and conditions which are inherently hazardous, irrespective of the fact whether or not the worker is a child or an adult are included in the list. While considering child labour, whether something is hazardous or not, should be considered from the point of view of the child. It is possible that any work even though inherently not dangerous, when performed for long hours without adequate rest becomes harmful for the child.

Some scholars also describe the spectrum of child labour, the different sectors in which children are employed as a 'continuum'. The continuum extends from acceptable forms of child labour to the most intolerable forms. According to the continuum theory each individual case will need to be evaluated. Generalist categorization is not possible because the same job may be very dangerous for a particular child in a given situation, but may be acceptable in the case of another child (e.g., Selling news papers in the evening by a young boy may be acceptable but not in the case of a teenaged girl). Thus child labour has come to be categorized as that of acceptable forms and unacceptable forms. There are other distinctions like the intolerable forms, the most intolerable forms and tolerable forms of child labour. ILO has accepted a new convention 'to target the most intolerable forms of child labour'.

This approach recognizes the magnitude of the problem and its complexities. It is pragmatic and utilitarian. But it attacks only the phenomenon and takes almost a fatalistic position that the causes behind the practice are perennial and unchangeable. This does not correspond to experiences elsewhere

Elimination of Child Labour

'Eliminate the practice of child labour' was the message of the ILO's initiative 'International Programme on the elimination of child labour' (IPEC) launched in the early nineties (1992) advocated. ILO and IPEC strongly held that child labour was not inevitable and therefore can be ended. Though it is a given practice today, it is not unchangeable. It need not be a permanent feature and it can be removed or rather eliminated.

The elimination approach targets the working children and considers it possible to displace them from the labouring situation to a schooling situation. It upheld the progressive total elimination as a possibility through awareness and action, first reduction and then elimination. This approach emphasized welfare programmes for child labour gradually removing them from employment. Such attempts were supported by creation of awareness and institutional mechanisms towards opposing child labour by working with trade unions, employer's federations, labour law enforcement machinery and so on.

Though the elimination approach gave due importance to education and worked with the educational system, it did not lay much stress on preventing the entry of children to the labour force through universalising elementary education. The approach was very close to an isolationist view, where by the phenomenon of child labour was viewed not so much in the structural context but just as a prevalent phenomenon. This can also be the result of an attempt to fully focus on child labourers.

The elimination approach was a short-term approach. It was anticipated that the practice of child labour could be eliminated from different locations within a short span of time without any change in the structural context, social and economic relations.

The elimination approach succeeds in defining the target groups and goals clearly. But it is a singular approach and is unable to deal with the complexities of this problem. While it tackles illiteracy and absence of schooling, one of the basic causes of child labour, other causes are neglected.

Abolitionist Approach

'Ban employment of children and make free elementary education compulsory' would be the main position of the proponents of this view. It is often argued that all the discussions on lack of alternatives; difficulties with rehabilitation, etc. are deviationist tactics. These are excuses put forward in order to legitimise and continue children toiling in all kinds of jobs.

This approach believes that children must be in school. Employers must be prohibited firmly from enrolling them for work.

Parents must be put under obligation to send them to school and the state must provide schools and access to proper education to all children.

The approach is fully political and the responsibility of existence of the practice is clearly fixed on the State. The State must act legally and socially on employers and parents and ensure the end of this practice. Others concerned like the civil society institutions must act on the State.

The approach sounds clear radical and fully political. It does not take into consideration the present state of affairs wherein a large number of children are labouring and the need to provide an alternative. Legal interventions can only be instruments for social change and cannot substitute it.

Eradication of Child Labour

The eradication approach can be characterized by its insistence on the search for the causes of child labour and striking at these causes. Child labour is viewed in its structural context as a phenomenon resulting from unjust social structures and inequitable access to resources and consequent deprivations.

Consequently, the approach has to be integrated, multi-pronged and leading to change in the predominant and social equations in favour of the poor and depressed. Child labour is yet another social issue or an attack within the on going struggle of contending classes and section for sharing of resources. The movement against child labour has therefore to become a part of a wider movement for social change.

Eradicationists would consider institution of free, compulsory and quality education as a necessary condition for achieving a child labour free situation. This itself will not be sufficient and has to be, however, supplemented with other factors like provision of fair/ adult wages, promotion of employment opportunities, access to resources through land reforms, removal of social and gender discriminations, etc.

In the given situation where a large number of children are already working they would endeavour to wean children out from labour and re-integrate them in the school system. They would embark upon preventing the entry of children to labour force by stepping up school enrolments. Improving the schools system and expanding the spread of elementary education when required as a part of the agenda.

Programmatic approach to regulate employment of children in certain sectors as an interim measure may be conceded while they argue that the employment of children under certain age (14 in India) has to be legally banned. Having a clear position to prohibit employment of children below 14 years in all sectors, the presently employed children cannot be thrown out into the open without any alternative. They have to be provided alternatives either within schools or otherwise. Regulation as a temporary step in order to provide benefits and give some relief to children under hardship or suffering may be acceptable.

The above is a point, much debated among those who stand for eradication. It is argued that any kind of regulation is contradictory to total eradication and therefore will be counter productive. This position is countered with the possibility of children ending up in worse situations than they are presently in, if not provided with an alternative.

Demanding adult wages for children has been proposed as a means towards making employment of children redundant. The argument is that as children are employed primarily because of the low wages leading to higher profit, if adult wages are made compulsory, the reason for employing children will not exist any more.

This approach of eradication does not view child labour merely from the point of view of the child. It places it in the socio-economic context, characterized by a large unorganised sector capable only of low wages, recruiting children in large numbers. Children are entering the labour force not so much because of their need and willingness but because of the large number of employers preferring to recruit children as against adults for reasons of low wages, pliability, submissiveness, absence of legal protection, trade union rights, etc. Hence a legal situation, which negates the possibility of employing children below a certain minimum age, is strongly advocated.

From the point of view of the families and parents, sending children to work amounts to exercising a practical and real option available, when faced with severe constraints of poverty, semi-starvation and a host of other problems. If such a possibility did not really exist they would be forced to look for other options. In other words, if employers were not permitted to employ children, child labour would not exist.

The situation is similar in the case of small employers running small enterprises. They too are faced with running a business and enterprise, in the midst of many constraints. If the option of employing children at low wages were open, they would naturally exercise it rather than look too hard for other possibilities. Such situations in the long run contribute to low wages. The low wages keep adults away from these occupations.

This approach enshrines that to defend the rights of children to education, play and leisure, it is necessary to have conducive socio-economic situation. The socio-economic status of the community from where child labour emanates should be promoted. Such a comprehensive approach provides several action points and leads to a long-term solution.

Product/Market-based Actions

There are some actions, which are of recent origin and are described as new strategies. These consist of creating consumer awareness about the involvement of children in production of consumer items and demanding a *boycott on such products*. The plea is then extended to traders, importers, exporters and also to national governments and associations of nations like the European Union or even WTO. This also ushers in the corporate activism against child labour. Intervention of trade organisations and corporate houses is argued to be very effective because such intervention threatens with real monetary losses.

Labelling of products as child labour free and thus attempting the removal of children from the production process is another form of this strategy. Labelling is a sort of carrot and stick approach as it included boycott of goods produced by children, while it promotes the marketing of the same goods produced without involving children. National governments and international fora like WTO have also appropriated such initiatives. The efforts of the American Senator, Tom Harkin to bring in legislation (viz. Harkin's Bill) were widely published. Though the Bill itself did not finally get passed, the US government has reportedly authorized the customs and Excise department to refuse entry of goods produced by employing children to the U.S. market.

Child labour also was a major 'concern' of the 'social clauses' in WTO which was proposed by leading WTO members some time ago. The protectionist interests of the developed countries were the driving force behind this concern on child labour, environmental conditions, standards of production, women's labour, etc.

Global awareness leading to creation of global political will against child labour is yet another part of the above approach. Tripartite bodies like ILO, UNICEF and other such organizations also play a major role in combating child labour. However all these are specific actions and reflect one or the other or more than one of the above approaches or positions.

The product/market centred initiatives may be seen more as tactical actions within other comprehensive strategies to end the practice of child labour.

The product/market based interventions and initiatives is in tune with the current market dominated socio-political situation. Trade organizations and trade relations have come to occupy a central place in all sectors of society. Economic planning itself is more commodity oriented rather than people oriented. Consequently such interventions have great relevance. However, the danger that such actions can be motivated by trade interests and hence be discriminatory to weaker economies is endemic. In the final analysis the logic of the market is competition where the survival of the fittest is the norm. In competition everyone naturally tries to take advantage of all possible options. The option of opposing low production costs and consequent market advantages to some nations under the garb of opposing child labour is an imaginative one!

Recommendations

Free compulsory education has preceded laws against child labour in many countries. An educated person is normally more productive and also healthy, as his/her health has not been hampered due to hard labour in early childhood. Thus poverty eradication itself can be seen as a result of eradication of child labour.

Laws for implementation of free and compulsory education in a way, though difficult to be implemented, are probably more practical than laws against child labour.

The view that parents and children themselves benefit when children are employed is a very shortsighted view. As argued earlier this not only harms the interest of the child but also keeps the wages low, the adults unemployed and productivity low.

While tackling a situation in which millions of children are part of the labour force it will also be necessary to have different kinds of approaches for different groups of children. Even in instituting compulsory education, it has been a practice to do it stage-wise according to different age groups, say 10, 12, and so on. Normally the age which children are allowed to leave school and the age of entry to the labour force matched. It seems necessary to have some age specification on this especially in order to formulate common policies and positions across national or continental frontiers.

The positive elements of different approaches of amelioration, regulation and elimination can be brought into the eradication approach and make it a comprehensive strategy for combating the problem of child labour. This strategy must include various tactical interventions. Care must be taken to ensure that the tactical actions positively contribute to eradication and does not block it. Such approach also provides space for different kinds of inputs and initiatives. The eradication approach may appear to be a very long term and complicated one. This difficulty can be overcome by formulating short-term tactical action points leading to the long-term goal.

In the Indian context, the age 14 years was adopted as the age of free compulsory education at the time of framing of the constitution. Subsequently the same age has been adopted to define a child under the child labour Prohibition and Regulation Act, 1986. Though the Act provides for prohibition of employment of children below 14 years in the hazardous sector and regulating employment of children in the non-hazardous sector, the acceptable position would be, prohibition of employment of children below 14 years in all sectors. Provision of free compulsory quality education for all of them and regulation of employment of youngsters who are between 14 and 18 years of age must be ensured. This would be in the spirit of the constitution of India. Within the given situation this can be actualized through a concerted action plan combining legal amendments and programmatic initiatives.

5

Conceptual Narratives in Human Rights of the Child Discourse in Developing Countries

I.P. Massey

Introspection, retrospection and self-correction are the hallmarks of any democratic society. There comes a time in the life of every nation when there is a time to pause and take stock of all the vital areas of national concerns. Today this time has come for India when we are at the threshold of a new century and have also completed Fifty Years of our independence. One of such vital areas where stocktaking is imperative is the area of human rights of the Child, which is a matter of vital national concern. Unlike the popular belief, in my opinion, child is not a 'resource' but is a source on which the future of the whole country hinges. The dictum "give me a good *child* and I will give you a good nation!' has universal Validity and acceptability.

Historical Perspective

Universal concern about childhood throughout this century has grown alongside the notions of human rights. The way human rights are now understood, especially in relation to child, has more to do with the individual's civil rights within a nation state, than with the universal principles of equality liberty and fraternity, known as natural rights, which were proposed in the French Revolution and later enshrined in the various constitutions of the world, including India.

Right of the Child is a precious gift of the present century. In this century a notion developed that how a state treats its citizens is *no* longer a matter in its own sovereign domain but is a matter of legitimate concern of the total community of the nations.[1] It is for this reason that the UNO through its various Declarations, Conventions and Protocols have set out norms and standards of treatment of its citizens including children. These norms and standards, so far as the child is concerned, are those norms and standards, which every civilized society should aspire for and follow.

The treatment, which a society gives to its children, is the most precious, but the most vulnerable section of its society, since, it determines the level of its civilization and culture. Viewed from this perspective, there is hardly anything on the basis of which one can feel proud as a member of a civilized world. UNICEF's Executive Director, Mr. James Grant, addressing the Executive Board in June, 1993 remarked:

> ". . . I now take the liberty, with your permission, of asking the Executive Board to observe a moment of silent respect for the 40,000 children who, dying this day largely from preventable and environmental causes, are losing their chance to enjoy the potential benefits and opportunities of Mother Earth and for the 40,000 who lost that chance yesterday and the 40,000 children who, will lose it tomorrow and every day. These deaths are not only the ultimate waste of the most precious resources of our planet, but as we learn how to prevent them, they are increasingly becoming an obscenity. Morality marches with the changing capacity."[2]

Another peculiarity of this century is that there is a paradigm shift in the area of human rights from 'recognition' to 'realization'. Today, people are not satisfied by the mere recognition of their rights. They want empowerment through state's affirmative action necessary for the realization of their rights and children are no exception to this. It is not denying the fact, that we have failed miserably in empowering our children, which is necessary for the realization of their rights granted to them in various national and international charters. This voiceless segment of our society continues to suffer deprivation, exploitation and destitution. Whatever running we have done has only been sufficient to keep us in the place and, therefore, unless we double our efforts it will not be possible for us to move forward the direction of empowerment of children. Reasons for this state of affairs are various and varied. However, lack of political wills, inadequate laws, ineffective or non-implementation of laws, corruption, illiteracy and poverty continue to be at the top. As a result an estimated 300 million children population in India between 0 to 14 years of age group representing a little over one third of India's population is suffering miserably and silently.

Generally, every country in the developing world pleads inability to execute affirmative action plans for the empowerment of children due to financial stringency. Inaugurating the Conference on 'Shaping the Future by Law. Children, Environment and Human Health' (1994 Dr. S.D. Sharma, the then President of India, said:[3]

> "It is noteworthy that just ten modern jet fighter aircrafts entail a cost of nearly 7000 million dollars—an amount equivalent to the entire year's budget of an international agency like UNICEF working for the child welfare."

Another outstanding feature of the present century has been that the rights of the child are no more contentious but have become a fact. At a time when Magna Carta (1215) was signed or French Declaration of the Rights of Man was made (1780), children's rights were not an issue. Law even did not recognise the separate legal existence of a child. They were thought to be as the property of their parents. Thus the whole concept of the right of the child is the gift of the present century. The concept of the rights of the child is associated with the work of pacifist Eglantyne Jebb, who conceived this idea while working with the Macedonian Relief Fund in the Balkan War. She was the founder of the Save the Children Fund (1919) and was the first to formulate the idea of Declaration of the Rights of the Child also known as Geneva Declaration, 1923. She proclaimed for the first time that, all wars are against children. This Declaration later became the basis for the Declaration of the Rights of the Child by the League of Nations in 1924 and the Declaration of the Rights of the Child by the UNO in 1959.

Universal Declaration of Human Rights, 1948, which established a universal concern for the Human Rights of the individual within any sovereign state, focused some attention on Children's rights also. Art. 25(2) stated, "Motherhood and children are entitled to special care and assistance. All children whether born in or out of wedlock, shall enjoy the same social protection."

1959 Declaration of the Rights of the Child by the UNO was based on the principle of "first call for children". It states in its preamble that "mankind owes to the child the best it has to give." This Declaration was later on converted into a binding Convention on Nov. 20, 1989. Convention sets international standards for the protection and development of children and making it a matter of international concern.

International community almost took three decades in converting the Declaration of the Rights of the Child into a binding Convention. This shows that the rights of the child were not in high social visibility area. One may also suggest that after the Declaration, convention was not necessary because it was universally accepted that "mankind owes to the child the best it has to give". Surely the truth lies somewhere between these two extremes. Fact remains that child suffering is human suffering over which child has no control and responsibility

Elaborate provisions of the Convention recognize seven sets of basic rights of the child:

(1) The right to survival—which includes right to life, health, nutrition, adequate standards of living and identity (name and nationality).
(2) The right to protection—which includes freedom from exploitation, trafficking, abuse, inhuman or degrading treatment and neglect including right to special protection in case of emergency and armed conflict.
(3) The right to Development—which includes the right to education, early childhood support, social security, leisure and recreation.

(4) The right to Participation—which includes freedom of thought, expression conscience, religion and appropriate information.
(5) Right to non-discrimination—which includes equality in the matters of protection and promotion of rights.
(6) The right to a discriminatory treatment in case a child is in conflict with law.
(7) Right to implementation of rights—convention provides the legal basis for initiating action to ensure the enforcement of rights.

Convention further underlines the need of international cooperation for improving the quality of life of children in every country. These rights have been supplemented by the various resolutions of the ILO regarding child labour.

Constitutional Narratives

Constitutional narratives of the rights of the child are provided in Art 39 of the Indian Constitution. It is a Directive Principle of State Policy. It provides:

The State shall, in particular, direct its policy towards securing:

(1) that the health and strength of workers, men and women, and the tender age of children are not abused and that citizens are not forced by economic necessity to enter avocations unsuited to their age or strength;
(2) that children are given opportunities and facilities to develop in a healthy manner and in conditions of freedom dignity, and that, childhood and youth are protected against exploitation and against moral and material abandonment.

Art. 24, granting a negative fundamental right, prohibits the employment of children below the age of 14 in any factory, mine and in hazardous establishments.

This Constitutional commitment is amply reflected in various policy statements (1972) and legislative measures. To mention only a few—Factories Act, 1948, The Plantations Labour Act, 1951, The Mines Amendment Act, 1983, The Merchant Shipping Act, 1958, The Motor Transport Workers Act, 1961, The Apprentices Act, 1961,

The Shop and Commercial Establishment Acts, (Year) 19__. The Bidi and Cigar Workers (Condition of Employment) Act, 1966, The Child Labour (Prohibition and Regulation) Act, 1986 etc. Besides these the Juvenile Justice Act, 1986, Indian Penal Code, 1860 and Child Marriage Restraint Act, 1929 also provide for the protection of the child,

Rights of the Child Discourse

It is significant to note that the signature tune of the Convention of the Rights of the Child is for protection of a child who is vulnerable, voiceless and defenceless and thus can just be a passive receiver. The potentials of the child as an active participant in the growth and development of the society are not adequately underlined. Countries in the developed world consider development of a child, merely a matter of 'quarantine of the childhood' and thus largely emphasise on the elimination of child labour or work. This creates problems for the developing countries where children start taking burden of responsibility from an early age due to socio-economic compulsions, which include avoiding starvation. There cannot be a better example of paternalistic attitude of the developed countries. Thus the image of a child, which emerges in developing world, is not that of an independent and acting child. The potential of a third world child is underrated.

Fact is, that in the developing world, poverty remains the biggest violator of the rights of the child. The problems of a child here arise mainly from socio-economic deprivation, which are the two sides of the same coin. In India, 73% of the child population is in rural areas where poverty is rampant. Out of this, 30% children live in the states of Uttar Pradesh and Bihar, which are economically backward. In the same manner 18% of the children belong to scheduled caste families and 9% belong to scheduled tribe families. As such these children suffer extreme form of socio economic deprivation. Therefore, unless the economic system as a whole improves, all talk about the rights of the child would remain merely a teasing illusion. The situation cannot be reversed by any trickle down method. Unless a system change is brought about in the international economic order and the rights of the child are linked to this system the child in the developing countries would continue to suffer deprivation and destitution. It is only economic empowerment of the parents, which can give meaning to the rights of the child in the developing world.

It is ironic that this simple fact is not being appreciated at the international level. Therefore, what is required is that the concept of the rights of the child is linked to the world trading system. Recently concluded multi-national trade regime (GATT), which professes to achieve economic development of all the countries, is based on the principles of competition and equality. One fails to understand that, how there can be a competition and equality between inherent unequals. Treating unequals as equals violates the basic principle of equality. Natural consequence seems to be unequal and uneven development of the world economy. Therefore, unless the emphasis is shifted from competition to cooperation, from equality to equity, from patents to transfer of technology and from free flow of capital to accumulation of capital in developing countries, poverty from the developing countries cannot be removed. Thus any discourse of human rights must necessarily include economic growth of the deficient economies.

At the national level, economic growth must be tempered with social justice. Fact remains that growth for the sake of growth is no growth. It is just a cancerous growth. This also demands a system change. Benefits of economic growth must percolate to the grassroots level leading to economic empowerment of the deprived and disadvantaged sections of the society. If one wants to help a hungry man he may be given a piece of fish or a fishing rod. If you give him a piece of fish you are feeding him for the day, but if you give him a fishing rod, you are going to feed him for the whole life. Therefore, unless a change in the system takes place, deprived and disadvantaged cannot be empowered. Until this empowerment takes place, the rights of the child would continue to be merely an academic possibility.

Human rights are divided into two groups—civil and political rights and social, economic and cultural rights. Civil and political rights, which are enforceable against the state, emphasize "freedom from" and social, economic and cultural rights, which are to be provided by, the state, emphasize "freedom to". Thus civil and political rights are not end within themselves but are means to an end i.e. social and economic empowerment. After the process of decolonisation is complete and almost all the countries in the developing world have achieved independence from colonial rule and have become democracies of one form or the other, the emphasis in the area must necessarily shift to social and economic freedom of the people. Unless it is done the process of realization of total concept of human rights shall never be complete.

A related conceptual perception, relating to the rights of the child, relevant to the developing countries, relates to the child labour. Righteous perception of the developed countries is that, child labour is an evil which must be prohibited, whereas in the developing world child labour is a by-product of poverty and hence a necessity to avoid destitution. It is the poverty of the parents that drives the child to labour and work. Under these circumstances, to follow the strategy of prohibiting child labour as an immediate goal would be counter-productive. Child labour would either go underground or would be diverted to still more undignified professions like beggary or prostitution. This has started happening where prohibition strategy is not equally matched by an effective rescue and rehabilitation programme. It is against this backdrop that one has to evaluate the legitimacy of 'social- clause', as an integral part of the world trade regime.

Countries like Germany have stopped buying Indian Carpets where child labour is involved. Such countries are going to introduce a trademark 'Friendly Carpet Action' which will deny free market access to carpets where child labour is used. Other developed countries are also inclined to follow the same prescription. Such measures have worked against the interest of the child in two ways. Firstly, it takes away whatever competitive trade advantage developing countries have in areas, which are low-technology and labour intensive. This measure has already increased the price of the Indian carpet by 5% in the international market. Thus reduced economic growth adversely affects the affirmative action plans for the child. Secondly, strict enforcement of such measures also work against the interest of the child, which goes underground and suffers still more exploitation or is forced into beggary and prostitution due to poverty. Human rights of the child should not be used as a rod, but as an opportunity and challenge by the developed world to save the child from exploitation.

Stark reality of the developing world is that, except in a few hazardous industries, not prohibition of child labour, but, stoping the exploitation should be the first step. The Child Labour

Prohibition and Regulation Act, 1986 is based on the correct policy of prohibiting child labour in hazardous industries and regulating it in other areas to eliminate exploitation of the child. However, due to ineffective execution of this legislative measure no significant dent on the exploitation of the child has been made. Even in hazardous industries, instead of prohibiting child labour, efforts should be made to shift the child labour to non-hazardous processes of the industry. It is for this reason that the Supreme Court, in *M.C.Mehta* v. *State of Tamil Nadu*,[4] instead of prohibiting child labour in match and fireworks industry, directed the transfer of child labour to the packing process, away from the main manufacturing process.

Even where, prohibition of child labour is essential, rescue rehabilitation mechanisms must be very strong to counterbalance the adverse effects of prohibition. Unfortunately, these mechanisms are either non-existent or are feeble. The result, thus, is more exploitation of the child and thus cure becomes worse than the disease.

The Supreme Court also in a recent Public Interest Petition rightly directed the state to create a welfare fund out of the Rs. 20,000 fine imposed on the employer of child labour, in carpet industry, and a matching contribution of Rs. 5, 000 by the State, to compensate the family of the child, against loss of income and also to rehabilitate the child in a manner, where he can grow into an educated adult, skilled worker, who is able to withstand exploitation. Unfortunately nothing significant has been achieved so far. The exploitation of the child labour in carpet industry continues unabated, as it has been forced to go underground.

Any human rights of the child discourse must also include a perceptional fallacy that exists in developing world. A child is being considered absolutely incapable of forming his own views and expressing it. This is so because the cultural ethos of developing societies puts premium on age. Therefore, there exist no mechanisms which allow direct participation of the child while framing programmes, policies and legislative proposals that concern him. This often results in 'mistaken kindness' to him, and programmes and policies become counter productive. It was for this reason that Art. 7 of the Draft Convention (1983 Draft) had provided:

"The states parties, to the present convention, shall assure to the child, who is capable of forming his own views, the right to express his own opinion freely on all matters, the wishes of the child being given due weight in accordance with his age and maturity."

However, this draft proposal could not become the part of the Convention of the Rights of the Child, 1989. There is a need that the right of the child, to be consulted on all matters that concern him, should receive recognition. The concept that child cannot choose and thus will have to accept the choices made for him by adults, has not helped in improving the lot of the child over the past decades.

Yet another significant feature of the human rights of the child discourse is, that trade unions have played marginal or no role in organizing child labour. The reason seems to be that generally child labour is employed in unorganised and informal sectors, where organization is not easy, but the political irrelevance of the child is also a factor to be counted. NGOs have certainly played appreciable role in this direction. The result is that no effective pressure could be built, compelling the government to frame right kind of laws and no effective programme could be organised against poor implementation of such laws. Thus child servitude continues unabated.

It may be concluded that as long as poverty and destitution exist in developing world, it would be neither possible nor wise to completely prohibit child labour as a first measure. Under such conditions, first step should aim at eliminating the exploitation of the child and saving his childhood. Prohibition of child labour as a first step would not be acceptable to a "large mass of people lacking socio-economic empowerment, though normative narratives of human rights discourse have universal validity and acceptability".

But realization of human rights must necessarily be contextual. This world is not to be divided and owned. This world is for sharing. However in order to understand this basic fact, one has to comprehend the essential inter-connectivity and mutuality of all human beings.

REFERENCES

1. See generally Judith Ennew and Brian Milne, The Next Generation: Lives of the Third World Children., Zed Books Ltd. 1989, Sieghart, 1985, p. vii.
2. The Right to be a Child, UNICEF, India Country Office, New Delhi, August, 1994
3. Circulation by the Indian Law Institute, Delhi, dated Dec. 7, 1994.
4. AIR 1991 SC 417.

6

Magnitude of Child Labour with Special Reference to the Girl Child—An Indian Scenario

Mondira Dutta

Children are the first priority, because the foundations for life-long learning and human development are laid down in the most crucial years of childhood. This is the time when, a small positive change yields long-term social benefits and even a temporary denial inflicts a life-long dent. Thus, the opportunities of early childhood development determine the present and the future human resource development of a nation. Till recently child labour estimates were limited to children in full-time employment restricted to children between the ages of 10-14 years. In 1996, the ILO Bureau of Statistics revised its estimates from 73 to 250 million child labourer, acknowledging the earlier figures to be a gross underestimation. The new figures include children between 5 and 14 years of age and children who perform invisible work in the informal sector. The truth is that the vast majority of these children are found in developing countries, although child labour also exists in industrialized countries and is an emerging problem in many Eastern European and Asian countries, in transition to a market economy (ILO, 1996).

In India despite legislation since 1986, banning the employment of children under the age of 14 in hazardous work, It is estimated that an average of one out of every four children between the ages of 5 and 15 is economically active. Some experts concerned with child labour trends in South-East Asia believe, that the proportion of working children has stabilized and is even declining in some countries, as a result of various factors that have militated against it, such as higher per capita income and the spread of basic education.

Statistics, on magnitude of working children in general, is lacking in terms of adequacy and reliability, differing from source to source in India. Information on working children in the informal sectors, or even those who may be attending school but working at the same time, is difficult to procure and assess. Thus collecting reliable data on child labour is difficult, especially because of the work undertaken by children in domestic and informal sectors are officially excluded from the category of workers. It is difficult to assess their productive value. Hence, figures on child labour officially are always different from the statistics quoted by non-governmental organisation. For example, the 1983 Operations Research Group of Baroda estimated the number of child workers at 44.5 million. The Planning Commission put the figure at around 20 million by the end of the year 2000. According to the National Sample Survey of 1987-88, the number of child workers was approximately 17.0 million (8.2 million males and 6.9 million females in rural areas; 1.2 million males and 0.8 million females in urban areas). There are yet several unofficial studies that put the number of child workers in India at around 100 million. This may perhaps be including all children who are out-of-school as well as child workers. Statistics from the National Census and the National Sample Survey Organisation in the country, which are government agencies, reflect the estimated magnitude of child labour to some extent.

The 1991 Census of India recorded, in the age group (5-14 years), 11.28 million child workers forming about 5.37 per cent of total child population. This was more or less confirmed by the estimates of NSS report (round 50th, 1993-94) which states 5.78% of children (aged 5-14 years) as both principal and subsidiary status workers.[1] The state wise proportion of child labour to total child population for 1991 is presented in Table 1. The state of Andhra Pradesh (9.98%) had the highest incidence of child labour followed by Mizoram (9.40%), Karnataka (8.81%), Madhya Pradesh (8.08%), Meghalaya (7.39%) and Rajasthan (6.46%). On the other hand the states of Kerala

(0.58%), Delhi (1.27%), Haryana (2.55%), and Punjab (3.04) recorded the least proportion of child labour.

The NSS survey reported high incidence of child labour (Principal status workers) for Andhra Pradesh, Rajasthan and Tamil Nadu. Insignificant changes in the proportion of child labour were observed by the survey for the other states compared to 1991 Census results. Proportion of child labour (both principal and subsidiary status workers) recorded high for Himachal Pradesh, Tamil Nadu and Andhra Pradesh, contrary to the general belief, as these states registered a less proportion of out-of-school children by the NSS survey 1995-96.[2] On scrutiny it was found that nearly 85- 90% of the child workers recorded by NSS survey in Himachal Pradesh were 'subsidiary status workers'. Similarly significant proportion of reported child workers were also of 'subsidiary status' in Andhra Pradesh and Tamil Nadu. This explains that children were doing part-time work in horticulture and agricultural activities for some time of the year, but at the same time they were attending schools. Himachal Pradesh has made remarkable progress towards universal elementary education. In fact, the education department in the state have adjusted school timings and vocation period taking into consideration the agricultural and other economic activity calendar. Thus, the concept of part time work and education can help in making parents agree to send their children to school, as is the case with Himachal Pradesh, provided there is easy access to schools.

The Girl Children

A typical feature in most of east as well as south Asia, particularly in India, is the continuous increase in the scale of discrimination against the girl children and the rising number of 'missing girls', which is in sharp contrast to the fact that there has been both a rising economic development as well as improvement in the status of Women in India. It is common in many parts of India to find girls experience the 'apartheid of gender' with her lesser claims 'decided at the moment her biological sex is known'. To be born female is not a crime, but one would never know it by looking at the deplorable conditions of girls in India. In fact, the rights and health of girls, from a very young age, are at risk generally everywhere around the world and India is no exception! Many of them are married and are mothers by middle adolescence, burdened with adult responsibilities. They are known to take on a major part of

TABLE 1

India: Estimated Child Workers (Aged 5-14 Years), 1991 and 2001

State	*Child Population*		*Child Workers 5-14*		*% Child Workers*		
	1991	*2001#*	*1991*	*2001*	*1991*	*1993 NSS (P+S)*	*1993 NSS (P)*
1	*2*	*3*	*4*	*5*	*6*	*7*	*8*
Andhra Pradesh	16655656	18107000	1661940	2364000	9.98	13.06	11.66
Arunachal Pradesh	219480	288000	12395	4000	5.65	1.43	1.21
Assam	6002474	7018000	327598	194398	5.46	2.77	1.98
Bihar	23585809	27062000	942245	836215	3.99	3.09	2.76
Gujarat	238729	385000	523585	340256	5.26	3.10	2.17
Haryana	7324150	10976000	109691	128397	2.55	2.53	1.50
Himachal Pradesh	4308223	5075000	56438	210825	4.55	13.03	3.00
Jammu & Kashmir	1241683	1618000		132554		5.53	2.55
Karnataka		9987000	976247	1171297	8.81	9.73	7.67
Kerela	11083831	12038000	34800	42203	0.58	0.70	0.52
Madhya Pradesh	5983926	6029000	1352563	1177918	8.08	5.86	4.46
Maharastra	16740647	20101000	1068418	911643	5.73	4.30	3.50
Manipur	18650065	21201000	16493	2675	3.72	0.44	0.25
Meghalaya	443212	608000	34633	14170	7.39	2.41	1.59
Nagaland	468560	558000	16476	5820	5.29	1.43	1.12
Orissa	174624	230000	452394	559599	5.87	6.51	4.89
Punjab	311307	407000	142868	118070	3.04	2.24	1.80
Rajasthan	7704761	8596000	774199	1564101	6.46	10.96	8.56
Sikkim	4702876	5271000	5598	850	5.18	0.63	0.55
Tamil Nadu	11992321	14271000	578889	949591	4.83	7.76	6.92
Tripura	107975	135000	16478	14806	2.29	1.62	1.62
Uttar Pradesh	11979383	12237000	1410086	1920887	3.81	4.45	3.15
West Bengal	719352	914000	711691	885950	4.16	4.63	3.31
Andaman Islands	37021048	43166000	1265	5663	1.82	6.09	1.20
Chandigarh	17105523	19135000	1870	000	1.40	0.00	0.00
Dadra & Nagar	69610	93000	4416	699	13.2	1.52	1.52
Delhi	133605	214000	27351	24244	1.27	0.83	0.83
Daman & Diu	33414	46000	941	147	3.89	0.42	0.42
Goa	24164	35000	4656	6737	1.95	1.75	0.00
Lakshweep	2145281	2921000	34	000	0.27	00	0.00

(*Contd.*)

1	2	3	4	5	6	7	8
Mizoram	12687	17000	16411	3266	9.40	1.42	0.71
Pondicherry	173610	269000	2680	3577	1.54	1.33	1.33
INDIA	209986630	242112000	11285349	13994073	5.37	5.78	4.51

Note: P: Principal Worker, S: Subsidiary worker.
Projected Child population is based on Population Projection Report prepared by the Expert Committee in 1996. The projected population for India in 2001 is 1,012,386,000. The recent provisional population figures given by the Census Commissioner on 27th March 2001, based on Census results of 2001 indicates India's population at 1,027,015,247. It shows marginal variation compared to the projected population for 2001 by the Expert Committee.

Sources:
- Child Workers 1991 based on C-Series Census data (both Main and Marginal Workers).
- Child Workers for 2001 was worked out taking the following inputs.
  (a) State wise projected child population 2001 from Census of India, Projection Population Report –1996
  (b) NSS data Round 50th(1992-93) depicting % workers (Principal Status (PS) and Subsidiary Status (S) among the children aged 5-9 and 10-14 groups. The % workers were also assumed to continue for 2000. However this may be an overestimation for 2000.
  (c) Out-of-school children were worked out on the basis of NSS round 52. (For Details refer: Zutshi, Bupinder (2000) *A Situational Analysis of Street and Working Children in India,* UNESCO Report.

caring for younger siblings and household chores even before adolescence.

Girls are socialized to put themselves last, in majority of the spleres from an early age. They are subjected to enormous work at home and in the fields. They fetch water, collect fuel wood; cook, clean, wash, take care of siblings and thus act like little mothers. Besides, they work relentlessly, in all seasons, as agricultural labourers. Several hundreds of girls work in stone and lime quarries in many areas. They carry head loads of sand and rubble from the pits, at least fifty feet down the risky narrow stairways. Patterns of limited opportunity and cultural expectations shape the lifetime potential for the vast majority of girls. This in turn has a cumulative effect that culminates into adult women being hindered, discriminated against or otherwise being put in a disadvantage position, having fewer rights and opportunities as compared with men. This discrimination and neglect in childhood initiates a lifelong downward spiral of deprivation and exclusion from the social mainstream, in participating actively, effectively and equally with boys at all levels of social, economic, political and cultural leadership. These discriminatory perceptions of the Indian community towards the girl child, are fairly constant across all sections of the Indian society.

As females and as children, girls are doubly vulnerable, they are helpless, the least protected and can hardly protect themselves. Environments that should be safe for girls like schools, homes, communities and families—are not much. Thus the situation of the girl child is a matter of grave concern. The 'mindset or belief that girls are more a liability than an asset', still exists in the patriarchal practices enshrined within the family structure of the present day society. Merely creating laws cannot wash away such a belief evolved through time. The excessive female mortality before birth, at birth and in infancy as well as childhood, all ultimately leads to an imbalanced sex ratio with the absence of many of Indian daughters who do not survive till womanhood. The girl children require special attention because of the gender bias and discrimination they suffer from a tender age in terms of education, nutrition, recreation and the development of health and intellectual capacity.

A study of Table 2 clearly reveals the plight of girls in the initial years of infancy. The age group (3-6) years and also during the formative years in the age group of (6-11) shows a steady decline in the percentage of girl child population over the decades. India with a population of 1.02 billion constitute almost 45% children, under 18 years of age according to 2001 preliminary Census information. The entire Girl children in the age group of 0-14 years, who are the most vulnerable and potential target for child labour accounts for 37.4% of the total female population.

TABLE 2

Percentage of Child-Population to Total Population Census Years

Age Group		*1961*	*1971*	*1981*	** 1991*
3-6	Boys	9.56	9.62	8.79	8.44
	Girls	9.88	9.78	9.02	8.57
	Total	9.72	9.70	8.90	8.50
6-11	Boys	14.48	15.35	14.92	13.73
	Girls	14.60	15.36	14.95	13.85
	Total	14.54	15.35	14.93	13.79

(Contd.)

Age Group		1961	1971	1981	* 1991
11-14	Boys	6.35	6.87	7.45	6.35
	Girls	5.85	6.49	7.12	6.17
	Total	6.11	6.69	7.29	6.26
14-16	Boys	3.95	4.38	4.83	4.44
	Girls	3.57	3.98	4.44	4.10
	Total	3.76	4.18	4.64	4.28
16-18	Boys	2.92	3.22	3.54	3.35
	Girls	2.93	3.10	3.50	3.19
	Total	2.93	3.17	3.52	3.27

Sources:

1961: Census of India, Vol. 1, Part II (c) (I) Social and Cultural Tables.
1971: Census of India, 1971, Part II Special.
1981: Census of India, 1981, Paper 5 of 1984 – Age Tables.
1991: Registrar General of India. (*) Excluding J&K.

It is alarming to note that even in the third millennium, the latest Census information for 2001, registers a massive fall in the sex ratio of children in the age group of 0-6 years. From 945 in 1991 it has decreased to 927 in 2001. The sex ratio for 1991 also showed a consistently low value for states like Punjab, Haryana, Rajasthan and Uttar Pradesh in almost all age groups (refer Table 3). The states of Bihar and Gujarat, in fact, show a decrease in sex ratio with the increase in age, which means higher mortality rate for the girl child.

TABLE 3
Age Specific Sex Ratio, 1991

1991 Census Data	*Sex Ratio 0-4*	*Sex Ratio 5-9*	*Sex Ratio 10-14*
India	955	938	900
Andhra Pradesh	978	976	922
Arunachal Pradesh	1005	936	917
Assam	978	975	951
Bihar	978	926	826
Goa	963	976	952
Gujarat	939	937	908
Haryana	887	880	845
Himachal Pradesh	945	967	955
Karnataka	962	985	971
Kerala	951	977	981

(*Contd.*)

1991 Census Data	*Sex Ratio 0-4*	*Sex Ratio 5-9*	*Sex Ratio 10-14*
Madhya Pradesh	967	952	896
Maharastra	946	947	922
Manipur	974	979	979
Meghalaya	990	988	985
Mizoram	980	996	990
Nagaland	1006	965	942
Orissa	974	970	992
Punjab	874	885	886
Rajasthan	936	902	877
Sikkim	965	1001	950
Tamil Nadu	951	963	957
Tripura	971	966	958
Uttar Pradesh	946	894	834
West Bengal	972	967	949
A & N Islands	977	992	915
Chandigarh	904	895	846
Dadar & Nagar	1004	1005	905
Daman & Diu	964	952	964
Delhi	923	903	863
Lakshdweep	960	922	924
Pondicheery	967	961	983

Source: Census of India – C-Series, 1991.

Reports unfortunately confirm that the practice of the two social evils viz. female foeticide and female infanticide, plays a dominant role in pulling down the national average of sex ratio even today. The strong preference for sons is responsible to a large extent for the ever-declining sex ratio. The special studies on the 'Declining Sex Ratio and the Problem of Female Infanticide' sponsored in 1993, by the nodal Department of Women and Child Development, New Delhi, have revealed that while the practice of female foeticide is a common phenomenon in urban areas, the problem of female infanticide is a localised phenomenon practised within certain communities in the States of Tamil Nadu, Bihar, Gujarat, Punjab, Haryana, Madhya Pradesh and Rajasthan. Misuse of the modern technique of Amniocentesis for sex determination is an added dimension to this problem. In fact, the present ban on the sex determination test through the enactment of the 'Pre-Natal Diagnostic Techniques (Regulation and Prevention of Misuse) Act, 1994, has hardly changed the situation. Adding to this is the problem of ineffective implementation of the Act of Compulsory Registration of Births and Deaths, which fail to provide information on vital statistics.

It is quite a common feature to find millions of girl children working as domestic servants in India, but figures are not available, especially since this is often not counted as "work" in any official estimate. Many of them also work under conditions of bonded servitude or are engaged in marginal and illegal activities, which are most difficult to enumerate and regulate. They include the drug trade, pornography, prostitution and the many activities performed by street and 'nowhere' children.

Although education is found to have been an effective means to redress child exploitation, efforts to making positive changes have been largely ineffective because of lack of adequate school system and financial resources. According to UNICEF, nearly 35 per cent of primary school age children in South Asia, are not attending school. The 1990 World Conference on Education for All, held in Jomtiem, Thailand, constituted a global recognition of education as a fundamental right and necessity for overall human and national development. In doing so, the meeting, convened by the executive heads of UNDP, UNESCO, UNFPA, UNICEF, and the World Bank, made a commitment to ensure that the basic learning needs of all children, besides youth and adults are met. This international concern and support for the girl child was an important contribution to and deciding factor in the preparations for the 4th UN conference for women held in Beijing in 1995. Here for the first time in the history of human, women's and children's rights, girls won an important place on an international agenda.

Although skills, knowledge, competencies, and attitudes are the essential foundation for lifelong learning, recognition to the fact that basic education extends far beyond schooling and can occur in the family, the community, and indeed, the workplace, goes a long way in eradicating child labour. The linkage between child labour and education must also be understood in the larger context of powerful social, economic, political, and cultural forces, which play a major role in determining the level of child participation in both activities. Economic, social and cultural forces "pull" girl children from school, while factors in the education system itself play a role in "pushing" them away. Schools may be too far away or too crowded, discouraging families from sending their children, especially the girl children, where safety is a critical factor. Inflexible school calendars cause large numbers of girl children in rural agricultural areas to drop out because they are forced to be out of school to harvest or plant. Girls drop out at a higher rate than boys because they are required to work at home. In many schools, resources go largely to infrastructure and packaged educational curriculam, which often ignore the cultural content of learning and its impact on children (Boyden, 1993).

Magnitude of Girl Child Labour

One of the ways to get a fair idea about the magnitude of girl child labour is to find out what proportion of girl children are attending school. It may not be absolutely precise, but nevertheless, it gives a rough idea regarding the extent of girl child labour existing in the country at a particular point of time. Table 4 constructed with the help of data from the Census of India 1991 throws some light on this.

The table shows, girl children in the age group of 5-14 years constitute 24.5% of the total female population. Out of this only 43.91 per cent are attending schools. This means more than 55per cent in that age group are not in schools. The state wise information reveal that this vulnerable lot constitute more than 20 per cent of female population in almost all states, who are on the verge of entering the adolescence ultimately culminating into the country's future womanhood. Among the states, which show a low percentage of girl children in schools are Bihar and Rajasthan where almost 75 per cent of the girl children are not attending schools. Among the populous states Andhra Pradesh registered more than 10 per cent as girl child workers and a low percentage (a little more than 40 per cent) of girl children attending schools. Madhya Pradesh, Karnataka as well as Rajasthan also showed a fairly high percentage of girl children as registered workers. The category of 'Nowhere' children is prominently visible in Bihar, Rajasthan and Uttar Pradesh. They are neither those, who are attending schools, or the ones registered as workers. They may be working in the informal sector as domestic help, agricultural labourers or maybe simply helping in the household activities, looking after the younger siblings at home. This is a highly vulnerable group who are aimless and desperately in search of greener pastures. Their involvement as sex workers cannot be ruledout altogether. This is a dangerous trend and needs to be checked immediately. Unfortunately, excepting for the state of

TABLE 4
Girl Child Labour in India (5-14 Years)

State	*Females -1991*	*Per cent Girls (5-14)*[1]	*% Girls enrolled in schools*[2]	*% Girls Workers*[3]	*% Girls 'No where'*[4]	*% Girls Actual and Potential Workers*[5]
India	403359778	24.95	43.91	10.76*	45.33	56.09
Andhra Pradesh	32783427	24.76	42.02	10.54	47.44	57.98
Arunachal Pradesh	399554	26.44	36.01	6.74	57.24	63.99
Assam	10756333	27.39	43.46	4.07	52.47	56.54
Bihar	41172374	26.81	25.93	2.93	71.14	74.07
Goa	575003	20.37	79.03	1.94	19.02	20.97
Gujarat	19954373	23.94	5.45	42.46	47.92	
Haryana	7636174	26.13	52.82	1.81	45.37	47.18
Himachal Pradesh	2553410	23.83	68.01	5.55	26.44	31.99
Karnataka	22025284	24.89	50.99	8.71	40.30	49.01
Kerala	14809523	19.99	85.54	0.52	13.94	14.46
Madhya Pradesh	31913877	25.22	37.82	8.56	53.62	62.18
Maharastra	38103717	23.65	59.92	6.63	33.45	40.08
Manipur	898790	24.39	49.35	4.34	46.31	50.65
Maghalaya	867091	26.84	38.64	6.54	54.82	61.36
Mizoram	330778	26.74	62.33	9.75	27.92	37.67
Nagaland	568264	24.46	49.55	5.74	44.71	50.45
Orissa	15595590	23.24	43.13	5.43	51.44	56.87
Punjab	9503935	26.94	59.17	0.86	39.97	40.83
Rajasthan	20963210	28.06	25.28	7.88	66.84	74.72
Sikkim	190030	21.29	56.38	5.38	38.24	43.62
Tamil Nadu	27559971	26.34	66.14	5.11	28.76	33.86
Tripura	1339275	26.40	50.42	1.96	47.62	49.58
Uttar Pradesh	65075330	25.70	28.00	2.46	69.54	72.00
West Bengal	32567332	26.91	42.31	2.68	55.01	57.69
Andaman	126292	21.94	71.35	1.22	27.43	28.65
Chandigarh	283401	24.20	75.37	0.55	23.98	24.53
Dadra	67524	23.66	30.89	16.06	53.05	69.11
Daman	49991	23.60	62.80	3.88	33.32	37.20
Delhi	4265132	23.60	69.07	0.36	30.57	30.93
Lakshwadeep	25089	24.27	80.47	0.10	19.43	19.53
Pondicherry	399704	21.41	78.16	1.05	20.80	21.84

* % Girl workers is for the age group (5-19) in case of India ,while for rest of the states it is of girls (aged 5-14 years)

1. Per cent girls in the age of 5-14 to total female population in 1991 (Source, Census of India)
2. Per cent girls attending schools to total girls in the age group (5-14 Years) (Source: C, series)
3. Per cent Girl workers (main and marginal) to total girl child population (5-14 Years).
4. Per cent girls neither workers nor attending schools
5. Per cent girls actual workers and potential workers.

Kerala, all other states throughout the country registers a fairly high proportion of such children. The states of Bihar, Rajasthan and Uttar Pradesh are some of the states with high percentage of girl children who are either child workers (actual workers) or are not attending school (i.e. potential child workers).

Table no. 5 shows the school participation among the girl children workers. This was based on the 1991 Census data. The data from the survey reveals almost a similar picture for most of the states, which shows more than 80 per cent working girls are not attending schools. Data shows that only in a few major states like Himachal Pradesh, Punjab, and Mizoram a substantial percentage of working girl children do attend school as well. Quite contrary to this is the picture existing in the states of Andhra Pradesh, Orissa, and Tamilnadu, where more than 98 per cent of the working girls do not attend school at all.

The 50th round of the National Sample Survey, 1993-94 shows the work participation of girl children in the various age groups (refer Table 6) for rural and urban areas in various states of the country. In the case of rural areas, the age group (5-9) year girl children contribute significantly to the work force structure as principal workers or main workers in the state of Andhra Pradesh, Karnataka, Tamilnadu and Rajasthan. If one takes into account only the subsidiary workers, Orissa, Maharashtra and Madhya Pradesh have significant preparation of subsidiary girl child worker. In the age group (10-14) years girl children from the rural areas are economically active as main or principal workers in the states of Andhra Pradesh, Karnataka, Maharastra, Madhya Pradesh, Rajasthan and Tamilnadu. In terms of subsidiary workers, the states of Himachal Pradesh, Jammu & Kashmir and the state of Orissa contribute significantly in terms of workforce participation.

The urban areas, in the age group (5-9) years, in the category of principal status, significant contribution comes from the states of Andhra Pradesh and Rajasthan. If the subsidiary workers are considered, then the states of Madhya Pradesh and West Bengal also get included in contributing significantly in terms of percentage of workers in the same age group. The age group (10-14) years, for principal status workers show an active involvement in many of the states, highest being that of Andhra Pradesh, Assam, Goa, Madhya Pradesh and Tamil Nadu. In the case of subsidiary workers this age group of girl child workers are actively involved in almost all the

TABLE 5

India
Girl Children Workers School Participation, 1991 Census Data (based on 10% Sample)

Name of State	*Total Girl Workers (5-14) Years*	*% Girl Workers (5-14 Year)*	
		Attending Schools	*Not Attending Schools*
Andhra Pradesh	855438	1.04	98.96
Arunachal Pradesh	7122	3.09	96.91
Assam	119848	4.46	95.54
Bihar	323167	2.73	97.27
Goa	2277	5.62	94.38
Gujarat	260578	2.14	97.86
Haryana	36144	4.21	95.79
Himachal Pradesh	33761	17.37	82.63
Karnataka	477606	3.43	96.57
Kerala	15438	4.60	95.40
Madhya Pradesh	688871	3.00	97.00
Maharastra	597276	6.98	93.02
Manipur	9510	5.79	94.21
Meghalaya	15221	6.12	93.88
Mizoram	8486	51.01	48.99
Nagaland	8720	2.40	97.60
Orissa	207171	1.37	98.63
Punjab	18962	10.74	89.26
Rajasthan	445168	2.59	97.41
Sikkim	2868	3.77	96.23
Tamil Nadu	299705	1.89	98.11
Tripura	6902	2.74	97.26
Uttar Pradesh	422504	4.99	95.01
West Bengal	224451	5.11	94.89
Andaman	416	26.44	73.56
Chandigarh	344	9.59	90.41
Dadra	2624	0.50	99.50
Daman	459	5.45	94.55
Delhi	3575	12.11	87.89
Lakshdweep	6	16.67	83.33
Pondicherry	897	0.89	99.11

Source: Census of India, Series C 1991.

states excepting the north east. The main focus being in the states of Himachal Pradesh and Orissa.

It is believed that, greater the education facilities the lesser will be the child labour component. This aspect was studied with the help of co-efficient of correlation, which was calculated for all states for the two main variables namely, the percentage of girl child workers in the age group of (5-14) years and the percentage of girl children attending schools in the same age group available from the Census of India, 1991, (Table 4). The value of the correlation coefficient was 0.341. Although this shows a positive correlation between the variables, but the low value does not reflect a strong bond between the variables.

It must be borne in mind, that the national census data and household surveys often seriously undercount the proportion of children who both work and go to school, because they only record the "first activity", i.e. School attendance (ILO, 1996a). Nieuwenhuys (1994) points to Kerala, known as a model of less industrialized countries for nearly-universal education, noting, nevertheless, that school has not seemed to liberate children from work. In fact, she says that one of the underlying assumptions of the education policies has been that children continue to work in their spare time to support themselves and their families. Their absence in the child labour data and analyses, obscures the extent to which a combination of work and school occurs and may or may not serve as an obstacle to learning.

As concern about girl child labour has deepened and spread widely during the past decade, so has the understanding of its relationship to education. In the girl child labour field, a serious lack of educational opportunities is becoming well understood, as a major contributor to the girl children's involvement in harmful work. Conversely, educators and others concerned with access to education have noted that work and a number of related factors contribute significantly to the difficulty of millions of girl children exercising their right to education or benefiting from it fully when they gain access. These include quality and relevance of the education system itself, cost, inflexible schedules, long work hours and other hazardous working conditions. The relationship between the girl children's work and their education exists on several levels. Whether they are in or out of school, work may absorb time, energy, and resources at the expense of their basic education. On a deeper level, work and

TABLE 6

Girls Child Labour Workers Participation—1993-94 (5-14 Years)

Name of State	Per cent Workers Participation-1993-94 National Sample Survey Data (50th Round)							
	Rural Females				*Urban Females*			
	5-9 Years		*10-14 Years*		*5-9 Years*		*10-14 Years*	
	PS@	*PS+S**	*PS*	*PS+S*	*PS*	*PS+S*	*PS*	*PS+S*
Andhra Pradesh	3.0	3.2	32.9	37.1	0.7	0.9	9.8	11.0
Arunachal Pradesh	0.2	0.2	2.0	3.1	0.0	0.0	0.0	0.0
Assam	0.2	0.2	2.1	3.7	0.4	0.4	7.4	7.7
Bihar	0.3	0.3	4.3	4.9	0.2	0.2	1.7	1.7
Goa	0.0	0.0	3.2	3.2	0.0	0.0	11.1	11.1
Gujarat	0.0	0.4	5.1	9.5	0.2	0.2	1.7	2.4
Haryana	0.0	0.0	1.7	6.9	0.0	0.0	0.4	2.5
Himachal Pradesh	0.7	0.2	7.7	27.2	0.0	0.0	1.1	3.4
Jammu & Kashmir	0.3	0.3	7.0	11.9	0.0	0.0	1.0	1.0
Karnataka	2.8	3.8	18.4	25.1	0.1	0.1	3.3	4.5
Kerala	0.0	0.0	1.0	1.7	0.0	0.0	0.4	0.6
Madhya Pradesh	0.4	0.7	10.4	15.0	0.5	1.0	2.0	2.2
Maharastra	0.8	1.2	12.1	15.1	0.3	0.3	1.4	2.3
Manipur	0.0	0.0	0.5	1.3	0.0	0.0	0.3	0.9
Meghalaya	0.3	0.3	3.7	7.0	0.0	0.0	0.3	0.5
Mizoram	0.0	0.0	2.7	5.3	0.0	0.0	0.0	0.0
Nagaland	0.0	0.0	3.2	3.7	0.0	0.0	0.0	0.0
Orissa	0.7	1.1	7.6	12.6	0.0	0.0	2.8	4.7
Punjab	0.0	0.0	0.9	2.9	0.0	0.0	0.4	1.2
Rajasthan	6.3	7.0	29.2	37.0	1.1	1.1	5.4	7.3
Sikkim	0.0	0.0	0.9	1.3	0.0	0.0	0.0	0.0
Tamil Nadu	3.0	3.0	19.4	22.1	0.4	0.5	6.6	7.6
Tripura	0.0	0.0	2.9	2.1	0.0	0.0	2.5	2.5
Uttar Pradesh	0.4	0.6	4.5	7.9	0.3	0.4	1.6	3.2
West Bengal	0.2	0.6	4.0	7.3	0.2	1.1	6.3	8.8
Andaman & Nicobar	0.0	0.0	1.4	12.7	0.0	0.0	0.2	0.2
Chandigarh	0.0	0.0	0.0	0.0	0.0	0.0	0.0	0.0
Dardra & Nagar	0.0	0.0	7.6	7.7	0.0	4.2	0.0	0.0
Daman & Diu	0.0	0.0	0.0	0.0	0.0	0.0	0.0	0.0
Delhi	0.0	0.0	0.0	0.0	0.0	0.0	0.6	0.6
Lakshdweep	0.0	0.0	0.0	0.0	0.0	0.0	0.0	0.0
Pondicherry	0.0	0.0	0.0	0.0	0.0	0.0	0.0	0.0
India	1.1	1.4	10.4	14.1	0.3	0.5	3.5	4.5

@: PS: Usual Principal Workers; *: S: Subsidiary Workers

school are linked by the complex, entrenched and powerful political, social, economic and cultural forces which require for their maintenance: a population that is uneducated, cheap or free labour and powerless workers. It is not only about girl children today. Today's girls are tomorrow's women, her future clearly mapped out in the stages of her life cycle. To ensure that life cycle doesn't become a vicious circle, all need to work together to stop the discrimination at its roots in the lives of girls. Moreover, it should be pointed out that the perpetuation of child labour is neither in the best interests of children and their families; nor is it in the best interests of the social and economic health and wealth of nations.

Poverty: Cause and Consequence

Poverty is cited frequently as a primary reason for girl child work. It is true that poor families have a greater need for survival or supplementary income from their children's work, although this contribution may be an over-estimation. In the light of what is now known about the role of the range of factors, including poor or inaccessible education, work becomes a more attractive option than school for girl children. Poverty that keeps girl children working also serves to keep them out of school. On the most obvious plane, a girl child cannot be working and in school at the same time; "survival," it is argued, must take precedence over "development," and the best interests of the girl child are weighed by the contribution she makes to the family and therefore her own survival, illustrated by the direct and indirect costs of school. It has been calculated that "free" compulsory education covers only 20 per cent of the total cost of schooling. Other costs for books, uniforms, writing materials, transportation to school, need to be borne by families (King, 1990 in Ennew, 1995; Munyakho, 1992). There is also the indirect "opportunity cost" of schooling, the loss of income incurred by a family whose child is in school rather than working. The higher the opportunity cost of school attendance in relation to a household's income, the greater the perceived need for the girl child to work. Understanding poverty as a 'cause' of girl child labour must include understanding that it is also a 'consequence' and that it is the exploitation of poverty that perpetuates girl child labour.

Nowhere are the links between child labour and education more evident than in the situation of girls who comprise the vast majority of invisible child workers as well as the mass out of school population. Doubly excluded as displaced, minority children, many girls begin work as young as five, performing unremunerated and exploitative domestic labour. They are hidden as servants behind the sanctity of privacy laws in the homes of other families and burdened by the numerous and heavy chores in their own households—which are often not even considered work. The low status of girls reflects the low status of women. Whatever the factors that create a conflict between girl child labour and education, they are clearly reflected in the large gender gaps in education. Son preference, early marriage, and inheritance and social security laws, as well as a multitude of other important reasons related to schools themselves—(safety and distance of schools, lack of female teachers, gender insensitive curricula, etc.) stop girls in their educational tracks. The true value and high opportunity cost of their work, combined with poor opportunities for skilled employment (Marcus and Harper, 1997) and the prescribed role of girls as trainees for a life, confined to domesticity and subservience, make their education seem a poor investment for many parents. In Rajasthan, the Indian NGO SEWA, was told by 200 women that they did not want to send their daughters to school after the first standard because they needed to train them in work at home (Burra, 1989). In rural India, a girl works for nine hours a day and an average of 315 days a year in the fields and at home, providing their families, an annual income, which at minimum wage would cost Rs. 2,200 (or approximately $ 63 US) to hire.

The situation of the girl child is a matter of serious concern. An adverse sex ratio, high malnutrition and maternal mortality rates, poor school enrolment levels, high dropout rates and low skill levels with low value work are indicators of a fundamental preference for the male child and a belief that girls are more a liability than an asset. The 'mindset' in the still existing patriarchal practices enshrined within the family structure of the present society, as evolved through time, cannot be washed away merely by creating laws or evolving developmental programs meant for the general mass. It needs a massive involvement at the grass root level, which not only has to include the women but also the men.

A better understanding of the push/pull factors that link girl child labour and education have pointed to the critical need to improve and diversify education, and to do this through systematic approaches, using a range of modalities.

REFERENCES

1. National Sample Survey, 50th round was conducted in July 1993-June 1994. A total of 564,740 persons were covered by the survey, covering proper representation of age/sex, rural/urban areas of all the states of the country. For sample design refer (NSS report No.409, round 50th, "Employment and Unemployment in India", Department of Statistics, Government of India, March 1997). The data is presented for males/females for rural and urban areas separately for the age groups of 5-9 and 10-14. Taking the actual sample size of children covered by the survey, % of workers was worked out for all children in the age group 5-14 years.
   'Working or employed' was for a person engaged for a relatively longer time (one year) in any one or more work related activities. Such a person was considered as 'principal status worker'.
   A person was considered as 'seeking or available' for work or 'unemployed' if the person was not working but was either seeking or was available for work for a relatively long time during the whole of the past year.
   Anyone engaged in any non-economic activities for a relatively long time of the year, he/she was considered as 'out of labour force'. A person categorised as non-worker or un-employed or out of labour force, but pursued some economic activity, was categorised as 'subsidiary status employed'.
2. Zutshi Bupinder (2000): *A Situational Analysis of Education For Street and Working Children In India*, UNESCO Sponsored Research Study.

Boyden, J. (1993), The relationship between education and child work. (Innocenti Occasional Papers CRS No. 9), Florence, Italy: International Child Development Centre.

Burra, N. (1989), Out of sight, out of mind: Working girls in India. ILO Review No. 128, (5), pp. 651-660.

Ennew, J. (Ed.), (1995), Learning or Labouring? A compilation of key texts on child work and basic education. (Innocenti Readings in Children's Rights). Florence, Italy: International Child Development Centre.

ILO (1996a), Child labour surveys: results of methodological experiments in four countries Geneva: International Labour Office.

ILO (1996b), Child labour: Targetting the intolerable. Geneva: ILO.

Marcus, R. and Harper, C. (1997), Small Hands: Children in the working world. SCF UK.

Munyakho, D. (1992), Kenya: Child newcomers in the urban jungle (Innocenti Studies Series), Florence, Italy: International Child Development Centre.

Nieuwenhuys, O. (1994), Children's Lifeworlds: Gender, welfare and labour in the developing world, London and New York: Routledge Press.

7

Primary Education to Eradicate Child Labour

P.D. Mathew S.J.

The Problem of Child Labour and its Effects on Child Labourers

The Constitution of India forbids employment of children below the age of 14 in any factory, mine or other hazardous occupation. Moreover, it is incumbent upon the State to ensure that the children are not abused and the citizens are not forced by economic necessity to take up work not suited to their age and health. The United Nations Convention and the rights of the Child, 1989 forbids the exploitation of children for economic reasons. Accordingly, children must not be engaged in any activity that can be harmful to their physical, spiritual, moral and social development. Besides, the Minimum Age Convention, 1973, of International Labour Organisation aims at a total abolition of child labour. Yet in India child labour flourishes. The problem in its nature and magnitude is complex and gigantic. According to unofficial reports about 40 to 100 million children are employed in industrial and unorganised sectors of labour. Twenty lakhs of them work in hazardous industries and another 15 lakhs are bonded labourers. Child labour constitutes 5.2 per cent of the total workforce in India. India has the largest number of child labourers as compared to any other country in the world.

Who are the child labourers? Child labourers are usual children from Scheduled Castes and Scheduled Tribes, OBCs urban poor and riots victims. A majority of them are girls.

In what condition do they work? A majority of the child labourer are forced to work under the most appalling conditions. The unhygienic situation in which they work in hazardous is detrimental to their health. A good number of children in India are employed in agriculture, sericulture, brick-kilns, and construction work, hotels, beedi making, carpet industries and match and firework factories, plantation and domestic jobs. Some of them are forced to work away from home, as bonded labourers, to pay all family debts. Instead of learning, playing and developing, these children labour for long hours, stripped off self worth, locked by illiteracy and kept out of the world of science, art and progressive thoughts. Case studies reveal a trauma so deep, that many child labourers are unable to return to a normal life. Many others die before adulthood. As a working child grows to be an adult, he is trapped in unskilled and low paid jobs thereby perpetuating poverty. The state of the World's Children Report, 1977, says that hazardous child labour is a betrayal of every child's right as a human being and is an offence against civilisation.

Why do children work? Because they are poor. Poor parents need their children's income or services. Large number of working children have illiterate and unemployed parents. They may realise the worth of education but cannot cope with the immediate loss of a child's wages. They do so, as there is no option or alternative, to ensure their survival. Deeply entrenched patriarchal biases, poverty, lack of proper schools, boring curriculum, illiteracy and unemployment of parents--all combine to push children into work. There are also a host of other social, economic and cultural factors responsible for the creation, continuance and perpetuation of the system of child labour.

Why do employers hire children for work? Because children are compliant. They are vulnerable in a climate of mass poverty and injustice. They constitute a cheap and easily controlled workforce. Their employment helps the employers to avoid collective bargaining and to take off unconscionable profits. In other words, children are employed because they are easier to exploit.

What are the consequences of employing children? Most of the industries, which employ child labour, as a major workforce, are hazardous. Various health ailments are seen among the child labourers who work in beedi, glass and handloom industries. Children working in gem and diamond cutting industries suffer from eye ailments. Child sex-workers are prone to various sexually transmitted diseases and AIDS. Increasing sexual exploitation of children has terrible effects on their growth. Poverty and deprivation force children to work and once they face the world; many of them are dragged into crime. Many of them succumb to the harsh environment they function in and those who survive are physically and mentally shattered.

Past Response of the Government

How did the Govt. respond to the problem of Child Labour in the past ? The government's response has always been to frame more legislations, earning India, the dubious distinction of having the maximum number of laws to combat this evil.

The Child Labour (Prohibition and Pegulation) Act, 1986, is the latest legislation enacted to curb the problem of child labour. This lists 11 industries as hazardous, because they are clearly detrimental to the child. These are beedi making carpet weaving, cement manufacturing, matches, explosives and fire works among others. The legislation, however, suffers from flaws. The Act does not have any mandatory provision for education or vocational training for working children. There is no provision for any standing committees either in Parliament or in State Assemblies.

Legislation alone cannot be a solution to the complex problem of child labour, because Indian government is credited for its tardy implementation of laws. We are not a society, which fears the law. Guardians of the law are found to be its violators and speedy justice is unheard of. Yet, comprehensive legislation can be a great help for the eradication of child labour.

Government officials are not aware of the gravity of this problem. It was neither an issue for them, nor they are interested. They, like traditional people, are conditioned to accept child labour an ordinary phenomenon. This is one of the reasons that they, have inhibitions to work for the eradication of child labour. The labour ministry published its own reports without being actually involved with child labour.

Compulsory Education Phased out Child Labour in many Countries

What is the real and effective solution to the problem of child labour? Provide free and compulsory education to all children up to the age of 14 years. America had many children working in textile plants, factories and coalmines. Child labour there was stopped by making primary education free and compulsory for every child and taxing the rich to finance primary education. The Emperor of Japan in the 1870s concentrated on only one welfare programme, with a view of tackling all other problems--he introduced universal primary education. Britain realised its importance and made primary education compulsory in 1870s. By promoting education they achieved both economic progress and a breakthrough in population control. Through successful implementation of this one single welfare scheme, they have removed the evil of child labour from these countries. It is also compulsory education, which phased out child labour in North and South Korea, Taiwan, China and European countries. They introduced compulsory education when per capita incomes were low and poverty was widespread. In Kerala where education for all is a reality. Child labour is unheard of.

Apathy of the Government in India

And yet why did the leaders exhibit a singular lack of will to make this successful in our country? Is it because it has not been our tradition to care the poor, the deprived and the oppressed? Professor Amartya Sen has stated so succinctly in this regard: "Education in one of the odd subjects in India, to the importance of which tribute has always been paid in theory and never much in practice". He further added "Despite his (Pandit Nehru's) continuous use of the rhetoric of education for all, Nehru and the party he led put very little emphasis in practice on universal education when they gained office. The implicit concentration of on a seamless unity for India might well have hindered a concentrated effort, to remedy the deprivation of the educationally neglected. But the eradication of the deprivation is not helped just by admiring the non elite and their role in history, while leaving undressed their real deprivations that continue into the present." (*Ibid.*)

The Vision of our Constitution Makers

Our Constitution makers had known that India of their vision would not be a reality, if the children of the country are not nurtured and educated. For this, their exploitation by different profit makers, for their personal gain, had to be first indicted. It is this need, which has found manifestation in Article 24, a fundamental right against exploitation. The framers were aware, that this prohibition alone, would not permit the child to contribute its mite to the nation building work unless, it receives at least basic education. Article 45 was therefore inserted in our Constitution, casting a duty on the State to endeavour to provide free and compulsory education to children.

Primary Education is a Fundamental Right

The judgement of the Supreme Court in *Unnikrishnan J.P.* vs. *State of Andhra Pradesh* (1993) SCC 645, is a landmark judgement which declared that every child up to 14 years of age has a fundamental right for primary education. This judgement has far-reaching effects on the children of India, especially of weaker sections. Free and compulsory education for children envisaged by Article 45 of the Constitution, if implemented, can be an effective measure to eradicate child labour, which prevents them from developing themselves as dynamic citizens.

Importance of Education

The Court held, in the above case, that the right to education has been treated as one of the transcendental importance in the life of an individual and has been recognized not only in this country since thousands of years, but all over the world. In another case, *Mohini Jain* vs. *State of Karnataka* (1992) 3 SCC 666, the importance of education has been duly and rightly stressed. Without education being provided to the children of this country, the objectives set forth in the Preamble of the Constitution cannot be achieved.

The fact that right to education in as many as three Articles in Part IV viz., Articles 41, 45 and 46 shows the importance attached to it by the founding fathers of the Constitution of India. Even some of the Articles in Part III, viz. Articles 29 and 30, speak of education.

Since education gives knowledge and knowledge gives powers the preservations of means of knowledge, among the lowest ranks is more important to the public, than all the property of all the rich men in the country. It is the tyrants and bad rulers, who are afraid to spread education and knowledge among the deprived classes.

A true democracy is one where education is universal, where people understand what is good for them and the nation, and know how to govern themselves. Articles 41, 45 and 46 are designed to achieve the said goal among others.

Right to education, understood in the context of Articles 45 and 41, means (a) every child/citizen of this country has a right to free education until he completes the age of fourteen years and (b) after a child/citizen completes 14 years, his right to education is circumscribed by the limits of the economic capacity of the State and its development.

Speaking for the U.S., Supreme Court Chief Justice Earl Warren emphasised the right to education in the following words:

> "Today, education is perhaps the most important function of State and local governments . . . it is required in the performance of our most basic responsibilities, even service in the armed forces. It is the very foundation of good citizenship. Today it is the principal instrument in awakening the child to cultural values, in preparing him for later professional training and in helping him to adjust normally to his environment. In these days, it in doubtful any child may reasonably be expected to succeed in life if he is denied the opportunity of an education [347 US 483 (1954)]." [*Unnikrishnan J.P.* vs. *State of Andhra Pradesh*, (1993)-I SCC 645.]

Reasons for Failure to Provide Free Education to Children below 14

According to the observation of the Supreme Court in the above-mentioned case, allocation of available funds to different sections of education in India, was not on the basis of priorities determined by the Constitution of India. The Constitution contemplated a crash programme being undertaken by the state to achieve the goal set out in Article 45. But what actually happens is, more money is spent and more attention is directed to, higher education than to primary education. In this matter rural sector and the weaker sections of the society referred to in Article 46 were neglected more. This policy of the government was against the Constitutional policy as disclosed by Articles 41, 45 and 46. Educationists and economists have commented upon this inversion of priorities adversely.

Gunnar, Myrdal, the noted economist and sociologist in his book Asian Drama (p. 335) made the following observation:

> "But there is another and more valid criticism to make. Although the declared purpose was to give priority to the increase of elementary schooling, in order to raise the rate of literacy in the population, what has actually happens is that secondary schooling has been rising much faster and tertiary schooling has increased still more rapidly. There is a general tendency for planned targets of increased primary schooling not to be reached, whereas targets are over-reached, sometimes substantially, as regards increases in secondary and, particularly, tertiary schooling. This has all happened in spite of the fact that secondary schooling seems to be three to five times more expensive than primary schooling and schooling at the tertiary level, five to seven times more expensive than at the secondary level. What we see functioning here is the distortion of development, from planned targets, under the influence of the pressure from parents and pupils in the upper strata, who everywhere are politically powerful. Even more remarkable is, the fact, that this tendency of distortion from the point of view of the planning objectives, is more accentuated in the poorest countries like Pakistan, India, Burma and Indonesia, which started out with far fewer children in primary schools and which should, therefore, have the strongest reasons to carry out the programme, of giving primary schooling, the highest priority. It is generally the poorest countries that are spending least, even relatively, on primary education and that are permitting the largest distortions from the planned targets in favour of secondary and tertiary education."

In its publication "Challenge of Education--A Policy perspective" (Para 374) the Ministry of Education in 1965 said the following:

> "Considering the constitutional imperative, regarding the universalisation of elementary education, it was to be expected that the share of this sector would be protected from attribution.

Facts, however, point in the opposite direction. From a share of 56 per cent in the First Plan, it declined to 35 per cent in the Second Plan. It started going up again only in the Fifth Plan, when it was at the level of 32 per cent, increasing in Sixth Plan level. On the other hand, between the First and the Sixth Five Year Plans, the share of university education went up from 9 per cent to 16 per cent."

The fact, that the upper sections of the bureaucracy, government and administration, which make policy, hail from the dominant upper caste groups, surely account for the deplorable neglect of primary education. The structures of our educational system, is an inverted pyramid with greater priority and expenditure on higher and professional education, which benefit the upper strata of society only.

Ways to make the Education more Free

Free and compulsory education, up to the age of 14 years, may not be the only viable instrument to do away with child labour. However, it can play a crucial role in eradicating it to a great extent, because, it will benefit a vast majority of child labourers who hail from the bottom rungs of Indian society i.e. Scheduled Castes, Scheduled Tribes, Other Backward Classes and Muslims. The development policies pursued over the past 50 years, have persistently marginalized these sections and their neglect of education is inseparable, from the overall callous neglect in the entire field of socio-economic development.

To provide them free elementary education, it is not sufficient enough to abolish tuition fees in government schools, schools run by local bodies and private aided institutions. Other costs of education such textbooks, uniforms, School bags, transport and food must be borne by government in the cases of all children coming from poor families.

In comparison to many countries, India spends much less on education in terms of the proportion of Gross National Product (GNP). Only a little more than three per cent of GNP is spent on education. The resources gaps, for educational needs, are one of the major problems. Most of the current expenditure is only in the form of salary payments. Additional amount must be allocated for the renewal of the system and for increasing infrastructure facilities in educational institutions.

While allocating the available resources, due regard should be paid to the words of the founding fathers in Articles 45 and 46 and the requirement for proper balancing of the various sections of education.

Supreme Court Directions

In the context of our reflection, on the measures to be adopted to eradicate child labour, it is also important to study the response of the Supreme Court to this vital problem and the direction it has issued to the states to implement the programme of free and compulsory education, for children up to the age of 14 years, as mandated by under Article 45 of the Constitution of India.

In *M.C. Mehta* vs. *State of Tamil Nadu and Others* (AIR 1997 SC 6991) the Supreme Court has made the following directions:

(1) Every offending employer must be asked to pay compensation for every child employed, in contravention of the Child Labour (Prohibition and Regulation) Act, 1986, a sum of Rs. 20,000/-.

(2) The Inspector appointed under Section 17 of the Act, to secure compliance with the provisions of the Act, must see that for each child employed in violation of the provisions of the Act, the concerned employer pays Rs. 20,000/- which sum could be deposited in a fund to be known as Child Labour Rehabilitation-cum-Welfare Fund, District wise or area wise.

(3) The liability of the employer would not cease even if he would desire to disengage the child presently employed.

(4) The fund generated should form a corpus, whose income shall be used only for the concerned child.

(5) The amount could be the income earned on the corpus deposited for the child. To generate income, fund can be deposited in high yielding scheme, of any nationalized bank or other public body.

(6) The State governments and the Central Government must add their own contribution to the above funds to help the parents of the poor children.

(7) If possible the State must see that an adult member of the family, whose child is in employment in a factory or mine or other hazardous work, gets a job anywhere, in lieu of the child.

(8) In these cases, where it would not be possible to provide job as above mentioned, the appropriate government would, as its contribution, deposit in the above mentioned fund a sum of Rs. 5,000/- for each child employed in a factory, or mine or any other hazardous employment.

(9) The Government would either see an adult (whose name would be suggested by the parent/guardian of the concerned child) getting a job in lieu of the child, or deposit a sum of Rs. 25000/- in the Child Labour Rehabilitation-cum-Welfare Fund. In case of getting employment for an adult, the parent/guardian shall have to draw his child from the job. Even if no employment would be provided, the parent/guardian shall have to see that his child is spared from the requirement to do the job, as alternative source of income would have become available to him.

(10) In those cases where alternative employment would not be made available as aforesaid, the parent/guardian of the concerned child would be paid the income, which would be earned on the corpus, which would be a sum of Rs. 25,000/- for each child, every month. The employment given or payment made would cease to be operative if the child would not be sent by the parent/guardian for education.

(11) On discontinuation of the employment of the child, his education would be assured in suitable institution with a view to make him a better citizen.

(12) A district could be the unit of collection, so that, the executive head of the district keeps a watchful eye on the work of the Inspectors. Further, in view of the magnitude of the task, a separate cell in the Labour Department of the appropriate government would be created. Monitoring of the scheme would also be necessary and the Secretary of the Department could perhaps do this work. Overall monitoring by the Ministry of Labour, Government of India, would be beneficial and worthwhile.

Strategy for Compulsory Education

There are certain questions regarding compulsory' education. Who should be compelled in giving education to children? First the State, through its responsible officials, must be compelled to provide adequate opportunities and facilities to provide education in a given place. It must also make the poor children and their parents aware of the legal requirements and the importance of education and persuading them to send their children for education.

Should the parents or their guardians be punished for not sending their children to school? No, punishing them will be tantamount to punishing the poor for their poverty. It would violate the basic rights of families in a situation, where they are already facing serious threats to survival, as a unit. However, there can be psychological, moral and social expulsions, without physical compulsion and punishment. When everyone speaks of compulsory education, a social climate may be created slowly in every community or village or panchayat, that the parents, however poor, are compelled by the social pressure to send the children for education. Depriviation of certain socio-economic benefits or providing certain benefits to poor, can be another kind of incentive to encourage and 'compel' poor parents to send their children to schools. They must be made aware that, the primary purpose of educating their children, is not for securing a government job, but to make them healthy human persons and responsible citizens, who would be capable of building their personalities, families and communities. It is a fact that child labourers without sufficient basic (life oriented) education, can easily become victims of exploitation and thus ruins their lives.

Strategies to make Basic Education Relevant and Attractive

The Education Department authorities and school authorities must be 'compelled' to make the content and method of education relevant, easy and attractive to the children. Innovative methods must be introduced in the educational system, where there is maximum participation of children in the learning process. A good number of children, from poor strata of society, leave the school because they do not find education imparted to them relevant to their lives. Therefore government must adopt new strategies to make the basic education useful and attractive. In this context the ideas of

Mahatma Gandhi are relevant:

- Human being is neither mere intellect, nor the gross animal body, nor the heart or soul alone. A proper and harmonious combination of all the three is required for the making of the whole person and constitutes the true economics of education. (Harijan 6-5-1937)
- By education I mean, an all-round drawing out of the best in child and adult body, mind and spirit. Literacy is not the end of education nor even the beginning. It is only one of the means, whereby man and woman can be educated. Literacy in itself is no education. (*Harijan*, 3-7-1937)
- Real education has to draw out the best from the boys and girls to be educated. This can never be done by packing ill-assorted and unwanted information into the heads of the pupils. It becomes a dead weight crushing all originality in them and turning them into mere automata. (*Harijan*, 1-12-1933)
- I am a firm believer in the principle of free and compulsory primary education for India. I also hold that we shall realise this only by teaching the children a useful vocation and utilising it as a means for cultivating their mental, physical and spiritual faculties. It will check the progressive decay of our villages and lay the foundation of a just social order in which there is no unnatural division between the 'haves' and the 'have-not' and everybody is assured of a living wage and the rights to freedom. (*Harijan*, 9-10-1937)

Fourteen States and four Union Territories in India have enacted legislation to make education compulsory, but the socio-economic compulsions, that keep the children away from schools, have restrained them from prescribing the rules and regulations whereby these provisions can be endorsed.

Need for Socio-economic Programme

We have to acknowledge the fact that the phenomenon of child labour is embedded in wider socio-economic and cultural structures, related to family, community, caste and class. So the solution must lie in more complex, multi-pronged, variegated and nuances approach. Such an approach will have to take into account the needs of different categories of working children. Education alone cannot be the one-shot solution. Working children must be seen as integral part of the families. So measures must be devised, in order to address the desperate poverty, which forces at least 30 to 40 per cent Indian families to use child labour as a survival strategy. The goal of primary education cannot be seen in isolation of the economic and social status of the children and their parents. The parents of the child have to be motivated and protected economically and socially.

It has of late been realised that, constitutional pronouncements and their recognition, cannot make any headway, unless their structural roots are taken into consideration for effective policy framework. So, merely passing and making legislation against the child labour or for compulsory education, is not adequate, other socio-economic programmes in the most affected areas must supplement it. It is important because the problem of child labour correlates to the low socio-economic position of the parents, where the parents are unable to provide food, clothing, education and other necessary requirements to their children. Therefore. irrespective of whether they want it or not, they are forced to send their children to work.

Other Strategies to Promote Primary Education among Weaker Sections:

- Primary education must be recognized as the fundamental right and state should take all possible measures to see that this fundamental right is not violated.
- Governments must increase the budgetary allocation for primary education, which is the key for abolishing child labour.
- Tax system must be restructured. More people must be taxed and the used money for primary education of children of weaker sections.
- Existing structure, like panchayats, should be made responsible to implement the scheme of free and compulsory primary education.
- Parents of children employed, must be counselled on the evil effects of work on the personality of a child and persuade them to withdraw them from work and send them to school.
- Poor parents, who send children to school, should be

compensated for their loss of income.

- Through anti-poverty programmes, poor families must be financially supported, so that their children do not go and join the workforce due to economic compulsions. Simultaneously, there is a need to address structural issues, like land reforms and restoring the rights of people over their resources.
- Children should be motivated by various means to attend schools. They should be given incentives. Employers must be persuaded to stop employing child labourers.
- Activists and NGOs must collaborate with government officials and explore creative ways to remove children from dangerous work situations and provide alternatives for them. People at the grassroots level must be encouraged to involve themselves in curbing child labour and promoting education among them.
- The UN convention on child rights, ILO convention on child labour, the Supreme Court Judgement on primary education, 1996 judgement on child labour and the Report of the Committee of State Education Ministers on elementary education, must be taken into consideration on priority basis which will tackle the problem of child labour on one hand, and the programme of universal primary education on the other.

Conclusion

In the light of the Supreme Court judgements on the universal primary education and the abolition of child labour, it is again imperative to look into the government policies with regard to the above problem. At the same time there is a need to launch a systematic movement, on the part of the citizens, for the recognition of the basic human rights of the child and effective implementation. All those, who are committed to the well-being of children, must put their heads together and assist them, for their good and greater good of the country.

As expressed by Myron Weiner, India is a significant exception to the global trend toward the removal of children from the labour force and the establishment of compulsory, universal primary school education, as many countries of Africa with income lower than India, have done better in these matters. This shows that, what has caused the problem of child labour to persist here, is really not lack of resources, but lack of real zeal.

I end this article using the concluding words of the Supreme Court judgement "We part with the fond hope that the closing years of the twentieth century would see us keeping the promise made to our children by our Constitution about a half-century ago. Let the child of twenty-first century find himself/herself into that "heaven of freedom" of which our poet late Rabindaranath Tagore has spoken in Gitanjali."

8

Child Labour and the Imperatives of Article 45 of the Indian Constitution

R.M. Pal

There has been a lot of man-made, often deliberate, confusions about eradication and rehabilitation of child labour. The simple proposition, namely that child labour, which is one of the worst forms of human rights violation, must be eradicated; and that it can be done through the most simple method: implement the provision of Article 45 of the Indian Constitution:

> "The State shall endeavour to provide, within a period of 10 years from the commencement of this Constitution, for free and compulsory education until they complete the age of 14 years (that is, up to class VIII)". Send the child labourer to school and the rehabilitation process starts. And it is the duty and primary responsibility of the State. There is no short cut, and there is no substitute for free, compulsory basic education. I, would therefore, concentrate on the right of the child in the perspective of the education challenge. But before I do that, I may refer to a revealing controversy between two well-known activists, from a recently published book, *Against Child Labour*, edited by Klaus.

I quote from both, without any comment. Let the readers draw their own conclusions.

Swamy Agnivesh apropos of child labour in India, says in his contribution in the book: "I accuse the western powers of hoodwinking the poorer countries, politically as well as economically, and their insincerity is writ large. They don't want to grip the problem and solve it once and for all. They are playing truant with the problem. They are trying to run with the hare and hunt with the hounds. It's a double standard game and therefore, I don't trust even the Western media, which initially, 1 thought, were doing a great service by highlighting the plight of child labour and bonded labour in my country". With regard to the much talked about 'Rugmark label' and the 'Global March' in 1998, widely reported in the West, organised by Mr. Kailash Sathyarthi, among others, the Swami says: "After the initial enthusiasm died down, we found that there were certain other motives . . . (with regard to) the problem of child labour in India . . . We got to know that it was the German government which has largely funded the Indo-German Export Promotion Project (IGEP) to bring about the 'Rugmark' Foundation . . . We grew a little suspicious . . . when my own colleague, Kailash Satyarthi drifted away from the mainstream of Bandhua Mukti Morcha . . . . Surprisingly, the vested interests started projecting him as the champion of the cause of the child labour in India and thereafter honours were poured on him . . . Our suspicions and our worst fears came true when we saw a huge march against child labour . . . The western countries helped him to raise the money, around US $2 million or more . . . may be it doubled subsequently. The ILO decided to promote it, because the International Confederation of Free Trade Unions (ICFTU) was supporting it . . . We have seen the game-plan through and we think that the western powers are out to sabotage the real onslaught against child labour exploitation. They are going to cash in this whole situation. They are propping up leaders, they are propping up NGO's . . . The American celebrities who participated, and some of them were here in Delhi, were not shown child labour in agriculture or in brick-kilns or in the stone quarries, things which are not exported. They were straight away taken to Jaipur. . . This made it very clear, that the intention of 'Global March' was not to fight the child labour in its entirety, but just to highlight child labour in export oriented industries. . . . Nearly half of child labour is in agriculture, the other half's predominant share, is in industries or activities which are not at all exported."

With regard to the 'Global March' Mr. Kailash Satyarthi says (Chapter 8): "We have been able to initiate discussions, debates and some sort of movement in many countries [other than India and Pakistan) . . . This was another important achievement . . . (Another) aim was to sensitise, galvanize and influence the whole ILO process of the convention of the worst forms of child labour. . . . The March was officially welcomed by the whole ILO-Convention. . . . The most important part is the implementation of the upcoming Convention". In Chapter 22, Mr. Satyarthi says: "People should feel that it (Child Labour) is a serious problem. If there is a culture shock, so much the better. I believe that we have been able to hammer this into the heads of the politicians, the bureaucracy, the common people and the parents themselves...we could not do more because of our own constraints. I would say that the part of a huge rehabilitative, basic education, is still lacking. It is part of the government programmes and policies. In India, we have not been able to build up a national movement for basic education. Education is the most important alternative to child labour and unless the former is made available, the latter will not be eliminated . . . regarding the foreign funds, we personally were never influenced by their agendas. Rather, in most of the cases, we have influenced their agendas. (However) I personally know several NGOs where the people believe that if someone is a donor, then that someone is a great person. When any donor comes, they virtually lie at their feet, touch their feet, surrender everything...".

Without imparting basic education to our children, no improvement in any field and no economic development, is possible. The corollary is that this atrocious form of human rights violations—child labour—cannot be overcome without the implementation of Article 45 of our Constitution, (which has been made part of fundamental rights by a judgement of the Supreme Court).

When I look around, I find that in my campaign (a campaign with grassroots activists which has now been started by Professor Jean Dreze of Delhi University) should be supported actively by all those who are concerned about human rights for implementation of Article 45. Though I do not have the privilege of having the company of many. In fact, there are not many takers for the implementation of Article 45. (We must not confuse the provisions of Article 45—free compulsory basic education to children up to the age of 14—with literacy programme, literacy Campaign, adult education, non-formal education package and so on).

I may add that those who maintain that, this social welfare programme cannot be implemented for various reasons and yet, at the same time, bring out plans for eradicating child labour, indulge in unalloyed hypocrisy. Child labour is, of course, a human rights violation. What I have been stressing, over the years is that, deprivation of basic education is also a human rights violation—equally obnoxious and atrocious, if not more. This second aspect has been almost totally neglected, both by Indian NGOs and those from abroad. Even when some reference is made by some NGOs to the need for basic education, it is being done, half-heartedly. NGOs have been concerned, rightly, with child labour; but they have hardly been agitated over non-introduction of universal basic education. They have never come to the street on this issue. Why? NHRC and others who are engaged in human rights education must investigate this. They might find that one of the reasons is, the middle class mindset, which would have taken this violation seriously if the victims belonged to their class, but almost all, belong to SC/STs, OBCs, the Muslim minority and girl children. And as such NGOs belong to the middle class.

Politicians and bureaucrats, averse to or unable to, implement a social welfare programme for the deprived sections of our people, know how to get away with it through the inbuilt escape route in the system. Over the years, they have perfected and legitimised the art of doublespeak and the language of deceit and arrogance, like George Orwell's four-legged dictator who quietly changed the original thesis of the revolution, "four legs good, two legs bad" to "four legs good, two legs better"; and from "all animals are equal" to "all animals are equal but some animals are more equal than others". Our political rulers and bureaucrats, justify and rationalise, non-implementation of Article 45 in the kind of language referred to above. Language of reason has been totally lost on them. I give below a couple of examples of such language, as also of quibbling and backtracking, which is insulting to millions of our illiterate people.

The first announcement made by Dr. Murli Manohar Joshi, an eminent RSS ideologue and present Human Resource Development Minister, even before the Prime Minister sought the vote of confidence in the Lok Sabha, that all efforts will be made to provide education to children up to class 'V' indeed, a "fresh" interpretation of the Constitutional provisions!

On another occasion, sharply reacting to India being called the "illiteracy Capital of the world", Dr. Joshi angrily retorted, "India has a very large number of literate people also. Why don't you talk about them? The literacy rate is 50 per cent, so we have about 48 crore literate people in India, which is double the population of the US." Victims of human rights violation and those who are deprived of basic education know why Dr. Joshi and his likes get annoyed when reminded that India's illiterate population exceeds the total population of the USA, Canada and Japan.

The mindset behind this kind of quibbling and false pride cannot be expected to implement faithfully this social welfare programme. So that a vast number of our people will continue to be deprived of this basic human right; and our country will remain deprived of all the benefits including economic development, social progress, population control, reduction in infant and child mortality rate, and so on.

Dr. Joshi and his ministry, seem to have evolved a new scheme (reminiscent of former Prime Minister Mr. I.K. Gujral's scheme of making it mandatory for all fresh graduates to teach at least five children for receiving the Bachelor's degree). It is called the National Reconstruction Corps (NRC) which is to launch the literacy drive. According to Dr. Joshi, "the ministry doesn't have enough money" to impart basic education to our children. Therefore, this scheme, boys and girls in the age group of 18-21, who have passed their 10+2 examination, will be employed to teach children and paid Rs. 1,500/- per month. (*Source: Outlook Magazine*, 6 July 1998.)

Two short points in this regard. One, since the minimum qualification for teaching primary classes is 10+2 pass certificate, why not appoint them as regular teachers and pay them the prescribed pay and allowances? (The obvious answer being the Government doesn't have the money! The government has not been short of funds for anything except the programme of basic education). Two, girls and boys having 10+2 certificates are not equipped to teach students of class VII and VIII--children up to the age of 14. So that the NRC cannot be a substitute for compulsory basic education as a fundamental right. NRC can be introduced in addition to regular schooling with full-time teachers, proper classrooms, and other educational equipment. Or, is it that Dr. Joshi has now finally decided to stick to his earlier announcement, namely, that primary education will be provided up to class V and not up to the age of fourteen? (Here again, we are reminded of Orwell's Animal Farm and the sheep chanting regularly the revised lessons "And the 'form begin to believe that these are the true lessons! They forget the original lessons all animals are equal" and "four legs good"!)

Dr. Joshi has decided not to introduce the Constitutional Amendment bill, making free and compulsory elementary education a fundamental right (which was moved by the United Front Government). He and his ministry feel that it is not necessary to make it a fundamental right.

This is further reinforced by another exercise undertaken by a government of India, Research Institute, the V.V. Giri National Labour Institute in NOIDA. It has prepared a draft bill, the title of which is "The Child Labour Rehabilitation Bill, 1998, an Act to Prohibit and Regulate Employment of Children". Note, it is to regulate child labour. Furthermore, may one ask, what has happened to the number of constitutional provisions and the 21 legislative enactments on the subject? Nobody, certainly not those in the Government, need be told and reminded that these provisions, as well as the 1993 and 1996 Supreme Court Judgements, have not made any dent in the Government's immunity from action. Such negative and futile exercise is undertaken because it is an unwritten and unstated fact that, illiteracy, which is limited largely to the marginalized section of our society, does not find a place in the agenda of Government's priority

I may add that even our founding fathers—the constitution makers—did not attach any importance to this social welfare programme. It may be recalled that originally, the Subcommittee on Fundamental Rights of the Constituent Assembly, proposed, that basic education be included in the list of fundamental rights, but subsequently the constitution makers rejected it. One member said, "Is this a justifiable right? Suppose the government has no money." Pandit Govind Ballabh Pant quipped, "It cannot be justifiable. No court can possibly adjudicate", so "this clause be transferred to Part 11 (Directive Principles)".

Although this committee had distinguished and self-proclaimed liberal and Gandhians like Mr. M.R. Masani, only one member, Mr. K.T. Shah had the courage of conviction and gave a dissenting note. He said that if a right to education becomes non-justifiable, it "would remain as no more than so many pious wishes". He added "if it does not become imperative obligations of the state towards the citizen, we would be perpetuating a needless fraud." Furthermore, he wrote in the dissenting note, "Once an ambiguous declaration of such a right is made (justifiable), those responsible for it would have to find ways and means to give effect to it. If they had no such responsibility placed upon them, they might be inclined to avail themselves of every excuse to justify their own inactivity in the matter, indifference or worse". Prophetic wards, indeed! No surprise, therefore, that the operative part of Pandit Nehru's famous 'tryst with destiny' speech was not meant to be implemented.

What is worse is, that even NGO's "progressive" intellectuals and activists like the Sarvodayist's, radical humanists and other activist-groups, do not place compulsory education at the top of their agenda. In April 1998, Mr. V.M. Tarkunde prepared a document, on behalf of the Radical Humanist Association, "People's Minimum Programme for Prompt Action by the New Government", demanding that "resources should be made available to provide free primary education".

Mr. Tarkunde does not consider "compulsory education" to be a feasible proposition become legal, reminiscent of what our Constitution makers said. Does he, too, like the HRD Minister, refer to "primary" education, as, schooling up to class V? This dilution of Article 45 by the Minister and others, cannot be the result of "forgetfulness". Mr. Madhu Dandavate, when he was Vice-Chairman of the Planning Commission and this subject was supposed to be an the agenda of the Commission, did not find time even to have an in-depth discussion on the subject with experts, not to speak of implementing it. The former Prime Minister, Mr, I.K. Gujral, dispensed with the subject by making an announcement from the Red Fort that the provisions of Article 45 would be implemented. His government's performance in this regard was limited to the production of a totally unreadable report, to make elementary education a fundamental right, and more importantly, a fundamental duty, without spelling out the responsibilities of the State for non-compliance.

What I want to stress here is that this is a typical middle class mindset, which has never taken Article 45 of the Constitution seriously? I may also add that without a change in this mindset, implementation of this programme will continue to remain a distant goal.

Let us also give a quick look at the report of the West Bengal government, a self-proclaimed, most "progressive" one (whatever it may mean). The State has now been ruled by a CPM. led front for over 20 years. The literacy rate of the Scheduled Castes in West Bengal, is 42.21 per cent of the total SC Population of the State. This ranks way behind that of most other states in India. The literacy rate of the Scheduled Tribes is worse 27.78 per cent of the total ST population in the State, again, way behind that in most other states in the country. With regard to, SC/ST female literacy, the percentage is much lower. West Bengal does not come anywhere near States like Kerala and Tamil Nadu in respect of overall literacy and education--it is in the company of Bihar and UP.

It is in this context that we must take serious note of the report by *Human Development in South Asia 1998: The Education Challenge* (written by the late Mahboob-ul-Haq, one of the best known economists of our times and Khadija Haq for Human Development Centre, and published by O.U.P.) The preparation of the report was promoted and funded by UNDP, UNESCO, the World Bank and a number of other international funding agencies. (It is sad to note that Mahboob-ul-Haq's sudden death in New York, soon after the report was published, was hardly noticed in the media in our country).

The report presents a dismal picture. I give below a very brief summary of the report and also a few statistics relating to India, which should make all thoughtful people sit up and work for a movement to compel the Government to implement the programme without diluting the provision of Article 45. Once this is done, all other problems like family planning, health care, economic development, successful management of local self-government and so on, will become tractable.

Summary of the report: South Asia has emerged, by now, as the most illiterate region in the world and the income poverty is no barrier to the spread of basic education. If Sri Lanka and the Maldives could achieve over 90% adult literacy rate, and if Bangladesh could make rapid strides in this regard, why can't India make progress?

Political commitment to basic education in India remains both faint and fragile. With the result that India has the largest illiterate population in the world. Many countries that are poorer than India have managed a much higher rate of literacy: (1) Tazakistan—real GDP per capita income 1117 dollars, and literacy rate 98 per cent; (2) Kenya—real GDP per capita income 1404 dollars, and literacy rate 94 per cent; (3) Vietnam—real GDP per capita income 1208 dollars and literacy rate 78 per cent. In 1994 India's real per capita income was 1348 dollars but its literacy rate was 52 per cent. Mr. Naik maintained this in a report prepared for the Citizens for Democracy of which Mr. Tarkunde was General Secretary.

So that poverty of resources is not the real reason for India's dismal performance in the field of basic education, as stated by both the government agencies, educationalists and activists (prominent among them being no less present than the well known Gandhian educationist, late J.P. Naik)

Even in India, there are some states, which have made rapid progress in this field, which in turn have ushered in improvements in other spheres like population control, health care and quality of life. Karala, whose per capita income is less than the all-India figures, has a literacy rate of about 90 per cent. The other extreme is that about three-quarters of out of school children live in six states—Andhra Pradesh, Bihar, Madhya Pradesh, Rajasthan and West Bengal.

In short, the report points cut, India is still first in the world in terms of the number of total illiterate persons. According to official sources, female literacy is 26 percentage points below the male literacy, that is, there are 91 million more adult illiterate females than males in India. About 35 million children in the 6-10 age group, do not attend primary school; 37% of primary school children drop out before reaching grade 5.

The report states, "India's problem is that, the task of providing elementary education to all children is massive. The task was made even more difficult when India spent only less than 4 per cent of its GNP on education and then devoted less than one half of this expenditure to elementary level education. Both, the low over-all spending on education and its distribution among primary and higher education, make it extremely difficult for India to reach the goal of universal primary education. The amount allotted to elementary education in India has fallen from 56% in the First Plan to 29% in the Seventh Plan).

According to statistics collected by the authors of the report, from official sources, vulnerable groups in India are often deprived of educational opportunities. The literacy rate varies from 90% for rich urban males to a mere 17% for poor rural Scheduled Caste women. SC/STs have a literacy rate of 40% compared to nearly 60% for higher caste Hindus. The enrolment rate of 6 to 14 year old Muslim children is 62% compared to 77% for non-SC Hindus

Let me conclude this summary by quoting the main thesis of the report: "Education leads to many social benefits, including improvement in standards of hygiene, reduction in infant and child mortality rate, decline in population growth rates, increase in labour production and an improved sense of national unity. It is certain that South Asian economies cannot hope to engineer a decisive breakthrough in development or to become the industrialisation tigers of the future, without a generous investment in basic education and technical skills".

Professor Jean Dreze and Professor Amartya Sen also propounded this thesis in 1995 in their book, *India . . . Economic Development and Social Opportunities*. What they wrote regarding the wilful neglect of this programme deserves to be quoted: "In India, both ancient and modern biases shape our policies reflecting prejudices of class division as well as of traditional cultures. The difficulty in getting, even left-wing parties, interested in combating inequalities in education, relates to the general social atmosphere in India, including the nature of the leadership of the different parties which takes some major disparities as simply 'given' and not particularly worth battling against in view of other--perceived to be more pressing—challenges".

Some economists hold the view that basic education does not necessarily lead to economic development. They give the instances of Sri Lanka, Jamaica and Costa Rica where the literacy rate is very high but the economy has not grown very fast. These economists maintain, therefore, that economic growth leads to widespread education and not the other way. Which means, in plain and simple language, that eradication of poverty is the precondition for implementing this welfare programme of basic education. This amounts to putting the cart before the horse, for poverty can be eliminated only when the people are literate. Even if we accept their thesis, for the sake of argument, does it mean that our people must remain illiterate, and that our children must be deprived of their basic rights?

These economists also maintain that government should not

be involved in education, both with regard to finance and provision of education. They do not take into account the fact that implementation of social welfare programmes is one of the primary duties of a democratic government. How can a poor country like India achieve the goal of universal basic education without the active involvement of government? The governments of Japan and Great Britain in the 19th century carried out this welfare programme and took care of the total financial obligation in this regard. The results are there for all to see. Today, there is no western country, which is not wholly or solely responsible for school education. The private sector cannot implement this programme; it can and should supplement, as it has done in Kerala.

9

Child Labour Rehabilitation and Non-Formal Education

P. Das Gupta

The Growing Concern

To-day the alarming increase in the number of child labour has become the most critical concern of the country. National level surveys, census reports and State level data on child labour point to the gravity of the problem . These sources put the figure of child labour between 44 to 100 million.

These are the children, mostly working in organised and unorganised sectors of economy. A good number of them are a kind of 'nowhere children'. They are either working at home with the family members or are earning their bread through begging, prostitution etc. Some are engaged in insignificant economic activities. Largely they belong to the age group 5 to 14 years and are presently out of formal school set-up.

According to some reports, the number of out-of-school children, is about 84 million. It is being stated that approximately seven million children are at the moment attending non-formal education centres. And the number of children enrolled in formal school is 112 million.

The Status of Street and Working Children

The street and working children are often found in the urban slums engaged in rag picking, helping owners of road side dhabas and tea shops, carrying heavy loads, working in cycle/scooter repair shops, selling various articles of daily use, attending to household works and so on. They suffer from worst kind of deprivation and denial - health, education, protection, food, shelter and recreation. At a time when they should have enjoyed childhood, spontaneity, freedom, games and study with peers, they have to toil hard in inhuman conditions for economic compulsions. Struggle for survival land them to the stage of becoming victims of HIV/STD etc, the killer diseases.

The sensitivity towards child labour issue has generated a strong opinion for evolving appropriate strategies for rehabilitation of these children. The emphasis is on providing a comprehensive package of education with components of health, nutrition, recreation and skill training.

Universal Provision of Basic Education

The child labour debate becomes more complex in view of Government's resolve to universalise basic education facilities to all children. These children largely belong to either non-schooled category or early school leavers. Some of them are just pavement dwellers or those whose shelter places are railway platforms and bus stops. The problem of elimination of child labour and bringing these children within the fold of education has thrown a number of challenges before the educational planners, social activists and various sectors of people concerned with welfare and all-round development of children.

Implementation of Child-Rights Convention

National Government is a signatory to the Convention of Rights of the child. It is committed to adopt adequate measures for educational, physical, emotional, social and economic rehabilitation of children from disadvantaged and marginalized communities. This is reflected in the Child Labour laws and enactment, introduced from 1986 onwards. Some significant measures stipulated and initiated at the Government level are:

- Creating National Authority for Elimination of Child Labour (NAECL).
- Establishment of National Resource Centre on Child Labour (NRCCL), in the V.V. Giri National Labour Institute, with the assistance of the Government of India and UNICEF. Announcement of the National Policy on Child Labour. Networking and collaboration with 300 NGOs, State departments, legislators, various social groups and International Agencies.
- Launching of Welfare Schemes by various ministries.
- A call to the nation by the former Prime Minister of India, for making arduous efforts for release and rehabilitation of children employed in hazardous work.
- Opening of special schools for child labour under National Child Labour Projects (NCL Projects).

Among the measures, the most significant one was formulation of NCL projects. This was an attempt towards visualising education as one of the basic ingredients of child welfare services.

The main areas of concern of NCL projects are:

- stepping up enforcement of Child Labour laws,
- non-formal education,
- income and employment generations,
- special schools,
- sensitising public on Child Labour issues,
- survey and evaluation.

It was visualised that the National Authority for Elimination of Child Labour would play significant role towards rehabilitation of millions of children, working under inhuman conditions of life. It has members drawn from different ministries—Labour, Education, Women and Child development, Welfare, Health and Family Welfare, Rural Development, Textiles, Finance and Information and Broadcasting.

Status of Child Rehabilitation Process

The support system, created by the government at various levels, presents quite a positive aspect of the concerned issue. The measures taken for the release of children, from hazardous occupations are significant. It has made it possible for a large number of children to come out of their endless miseries and deprivation. However, inherent flaws in the Child Labour Act (Prohibition and regulation), 1986 has failed to provide relief to the large number of children, who are engaged in work situations outside those listed industries. Further, a section of children engaged in assisting their family members in craft activities also fall outside the purview of this Act.

At some places, it has been observed that, the policies and schemes failed to relate to the socio-economic realities of families of the affected children. For many households children work, not only to meet their own basic needs, but also for the survival of their family members. In the absence of proper support from the State and the society, such hasty steps have gone against the 'Right to Survival' and 'best interests of the child'.

Alternate Report India (1998), in this context, has raised some points on the Rights of Child, which need close analysis. It reported that, the Act has proved to be inadequate and ineffective. It does not require the employer to get a licence or permit to employ child labour ... It would have been helpful if a provision to this effect in the employment of Children Act was retained .... This would have made detection of child Labour easier and acted as a deterrent on factory owners employing children in hazardous industries.

Another important revelation, made by the report, indicates lack of seriousness on the part of some states in implementing Child Labour Act. According to the report, the ground level situations clearly point out that many states have framed no rules under the Child Labour Act to make it effective. No separate machinery, for enforcement of the Act, was created. Many states have shown no action under the Act. These factors have deeper relevance for the implementing agencies. It calls for identification of some viable strategies for effective implementation of Rights of the Child in the true spirit of the Convention.

NCL Special Schools and Child Labour Rehabilitation

Special school programmes offer different intervention

strategies for child labour rehabilitation. The focus points of the educational programmes are:

- Creation of a child friendly environment in the school for its spontaneous development.
- Provision of learning experience and conducive environment for emotional and social rehabilitation of the child. Creation of health care and nutritional facilities
- Extension of skill training facilities in the form of work experience activities.
- Generation of opportunities for continuation of educational pursuits through alternative channels - formal school, open school and technical training centre.

The NCL special schools thus combine the fourfold objectives of physical, emotional, social and economic rehabilitation of the child, withdrawn from hazardous industries. In the programme delivery community, people provide meaningful support to the school. The success stories have drawn many children from the neighbourhood to avail the opportunities extended by the functional educational programmes of these schools.

Non-Formal Education Programme and Child Rehabilitation Target Group, Focus and Coverage

Non-formal education programme has emerged as an alternative educational mode, to address the educational needs of out-of-school and non-schooled children. Its target groups are children mainly in the age group 6-14 years that, due to limiting conditions of life, are unable to avail educational facilities provided through formal school set-up.

The programme focuses on specially disadvantaged areas like urban slums, hilly terrains, desert areas and far-flung habitations with high concentration of street and working children.

Presently over 70 lakhs children in 21 States/Union Territories are availing educational facilities through 2.80 lakhs NFE Centres. 1.80 lakhs centres are exclusively for girls. 750 NGOs are supplementing the governmental efforts by running about 38,000 NFE centres, that are essentially in response to meeting the basic needs of special categories of children.

Ministries of Human Resource Development, Social Justice and

Empowerment and Labour Ministry, are sponsoring these programmes. Some international donor agencies are also extending financial support for child labour rehabilitation.

The child labour rehabilitation inputs are ingrained in the education designs and transactional strategies evolved under NFE Innovative and Experimental projects of Universalisation of Primary Education (UPE).

Special Features of NFE

Essential features of Non-formal Education (NFE) are:

- The programme, content and methodology are planned in a way to provide education to the child through life, for life and in life.
- It is in response to the child in the community as he/she is and is likely to be in future.
- Living, learning and working situations are fused creatively for facilitating child's physical, social, mental and economic rehabilitation.
- Participation in variety of joyful activities, within the learning centres, extends to that of community life outside the school.
- Transactional strategies are characterised by non-conventional and participatory modes of teaching - learning process.

All these components facilitate sharing of learning experiences and growing up together in a congenial and supportive environment.

Newer Dimensions of Child Labour Rehabilitation Process

The existing NFE and Alternative Schooling Programmes present two broad trends of rehabilitation process. The first category includes a cluster of agencies whose thrust areas are health, nutrition childcare, literacy, numeracy, environmental awareness, cultural and recreational activities, skill training, community service etc. Some also provide opportunities for participation in income generating programmes.

The other category represents quite a good number of NGOs

and voluntary organisations who, besides rendering the above mentioned services, have widened their areas of operation by opening Night Shelters, Foster Homes for street and working children and Observation Homes for juvenile delinquents. Further, these organisations are also helping children-in-high-risk through their counselling and guidance services. These cover both occupational, personal and health related problems including HIV/STD etc.

These 'walk-in' and 'drop-in' counselling centres are gradually becoming popular among the working children. Moreover, many of the NFE completers have got chances to work as 'Educators' for the vulnerable group of children. These programmes have, indeed, generated some hope amongst a large section of deprived and neglected children to look for a better life.

The programme packages aim at helping these children, to acquire basic life skills, that empower them with the abilities to handle problems encountered in every day life situations. The focus is to help the children-in-distress to improve their life styles in positive direction.

Challenges before NFE

The interventions initiated by various organisations, have gone a long way, in generating effective strategies for grappling with the vexed child labour issues. However, in recent times a number of challenges are being confronted by NFE sector. These are:

- Administrative and technical problems in mainstreaming of children.
- Negative effects on the children due to non-supporting learning environment of formal schools.
- A section of community people perceiving NFE as a supportive system for continuation of child labour phenomenon.
- Poor academic attainment of children resulting into loss of faith in the quality of NFE programme.

During the ninth five-year plan, NFE is being reorganised and revitalised in all respects - academic, infrastructural and management pattern.

Tasks Ahead

A number of tasks that need immediate attention are:

- Comprehensive benchmark survey of all categories of children, especially those working in unorganised sectors.
- Intensive community education programme, especially education of family members of working children on Rights of the Child.
- Creation of appropriate mechanism on a priority basis for monitoring the implementation activities at the State level and attending to the problems identified.
- Extension of existing health and welfare services of the municipal bodies to the street and working children, at a location and time suitable for them
- Creation of a special cell in the municipality for protection and rehabilitation of girls in the street, railway platforms, interstate bus stops etc: who are the victims of sex abuses.
- Opening of Seva Kendras (Service Centres) in the rural sector where working children with some skill training can be absorbed for minor repair work of pump-set, tube-well, fodder cutter, flour grinder, spiller, thresher etc.
- Setting up tailoring and canning centres for girls and establishing pre-school teachers training centres, for training of girls in pre-school education.
- Starting more number of shelter Homes for street and working children.
- Comprehensive documentation of process based success stories of Child Labour and of agencies dealing with the area by NCERT, NBT, National Resource Centre on Child Labour, VVGNLI, New Delhi, Mass and Electronic Media and utilisation of these material in the training programme for functionaries.
- Preparation of area-specific, occupation specific and working children's family specific work oriented intervention strategies.
- Adoption of holistic approach based strategies for tackling issues related to Child Labour.
- Intensive involvement of NGOs, VAs and community people right from the policy formulation to implementation stages not as mere partners but for generating new ideas.

10

Child Labour: NGOs Experiences

Ramakant Rai and Kuldeep Narain Maurya

Perspectives

The modem-civilized world has developed many tools and social indicators for measuring the civilizations as developed, under developed and developing in socio-economic terms. Perhaps, there cannot be a social indicator of civilization, that can measure the insensibility of its people, when the civilization becomes insensible than animals, by treating their children like commodities. In case of animals they properly nourish and train their children to become self-dependent. They take care of their children during childhood to make them fit for *"Survival of the Fittest"* society. None of us might have ever come across any example where animals have expected their children to feed their parents. It is the one and only, the so-called human being, developed and civilized creature on this earth, to exploit the children for satisfying their greed. Perhaps we are the biggest child labour employers in the globe. We inherit the ideals of "Non-Violence" from Mahatma Gandhi and 50 years back, the nicely spelt constitution regarding ensuring the education, health and childhood rights for our children, but are still fighting with the statistics regarding number of child labours (Servitude) in India. The recent Hon'ble Supreme Court's judgment, for the plight of children, has also become toothless. It is a matter of great concern that an effort during last government to make "Education" a fundamental right and thereby proposed 83rd amendment in the constitution, was turned down with the argument that making education a fundamental right will require 40000 crores of rupees which this government cannot afford. Surprisingly, the same government can afford to make "Pokhhran Test' and organise beauty contests, can save tons of rupees on saving Taj, Charminar and keeping cities beautified to attract tourists. Now is the time to introspect our government, our constitutional guarantees and international commitments, through various summits and convention, for the rights of our children.

Perspectives related to the rehabilitation of child labour are bedevilled a farrago of distortions, half-truths, skulduggery and veracity. The best crescendo initiatives often go away. Though the governmental line of thought, policy and mindset, keeps the NGO's at the thin end of the wedge, NGO's themselves toe the official line. Pessimistically, resigning to accept that child labour will remain and continue, and that the poor countries cannot eliminated it entirely but can be corrected upto a certain degree by throwing crumbs of basic so called service to the exploited, ravaged, deprived and forgotten boy or girl shackled to servitude for the life in highly damaging harmful and hazardous work environment. Let us ruminate the child, from whom the parents, the civil society, the private sector and the government snatched away his/her childhood, throttled his/her fundamental rights of education, security and participation. The child who is locked to toil for 72 to 96 hours at a stretch in glass factories among deadly, dangerous fumes and gases. The child who is doomed to miserable, extremely painful death from silicosis much before reaching the age of 13 to 14 years in Silica/slate mines or the girl left on innumerable alleys and footpaths of this country to sell her timid, tender, malnourished body for pittance. Let us surreptitiously think about the damage and destruction that we have inflicted on a child labourer's innocence, vision, dreams, personality, body and soul. And we have the temerity to offer and ask the child to come and attend a school for 2,3 hours when his/her days job is done? Is it not rhetoric of adding insult to injury to give a loaf of bread and a cup of dalia to raise his/her level of nutrition? When his entire physiognomy is blasted with fatal irrevocable diseases, disability and injuries, how far is it rational to provide health-check up, medicines or send him to FRUs?

Therefore, in our view, we suggest some points for consideration for development of a correct perspective as regards to the rehabilitation of the child labour.

1. We have to think, study, analyse and plan in HOLISTIC context. To lament, to shed tears and or to adopt vituperative strategy, to half hearted rehabilitation efforts will not suffice. We have to refer back to the world declaration and to the plan of action from the world summit for children, calling for promoting children's rights and improving their living conditions. The end-decade overview report, released by the U.N., depicts, a gory and startling picture. The economic crisis and macro economic shocks have led to an increase in poverty and disparity and left millions of people without access to basic social services or with access to services inadequate in quality. Economic growth rate is slowed by 1.6%, per capita income gone down from 12 to 3% and average longevity reduced up to 10 years due to onslaught of HIV/AIDS. Indian scenario is further grim and tardy. It is essential to assess the situation of all groups of children, identify those left un-reached and provide priority attention to poverty alleviation programmes

2. The scope of rehabilitation in addition to be taken into HOLISTIC context, it is further imperative to augment and broaden its horizon. The experiences gained by the NGO's in this regard need to be collected, collated and presented to the policy makers. Centralized action on the child and parents, does not bear sustainable impact. Therefore, it is necessary to address it into its entire perspective and gamut, including the community, the civil society, service-delivery infra-structure administration and political will/ commitment should be added.

3. In order to accomplish our goal, it is further necessary to desegregate the data to identify and reduce prevailing geographic, ethnic, economic, social and gender disparities.

4. Guided by the best interest of child it is imperative to promote a multi-disciplinary and cross-sectoral perspective in the adoption of policies, programmes and activities to improve the situation of rehabilitation work.

5. Building on the experiences, gained by the NGO's regarding child labour as a whole, it is of vital importance to undertake

Multi-Indicator Cluster Surveys (MICS) covering and dovetailing the demographic and health surveys and also harmonizing with other surveys, liable to be undertaken in days to come.

6. To monitor and assess the impact of rehabilitation undertaken so far, there is a great need for development of a set of indicators towards the health, education and mid welfare goals set thereof. New indicators to fill critical gaps relating to other areas of children's rights such as child labour itself, birth registration, disability accruing out of it, alternative family care, growth and development will also have to be worked out.

7. Some progress has been made in context with child labour. India has ratified a number of universal declarations and conventions and initiated programmes/activities to eliminate child labour like the global march against child labour and ILO conference, under which we are obligated to promote and achieve the effective eliminative of child labour. Hon'ble supreme court also took the historic initiative in December 1997 judgment. To ensure implementation of these directions, government conducted a survey (though the survey proved to be a big farce!). The goal of keeping the promises to the children requires acceleration, based upon firm political commitments to the realization of children's rights from the government, civil society, the private sector and the community.

8. There are a vast maiden areas of child labour which have been grossly overlooked and not taken into consideration. More than 80% of the jobs are hazardous with work environment and production process, which are harmful to child's physical and mental health. These areas are domestic, agricultural and unregulated (carpentry, repairs, iron smithy, weaving/embroidery), small scale industrial enterprises. Our concern and consideration should cover these areas also.

9. The myth that public is insensitive to the problem of child labour is not true. We have organised several marches from one corner of the country to the other. While, thus traversing the land of our country, we have found tremendous enthusiasm in the people regarding the child labour. School children are the best-motivated and enthused lot. The need is to tap these resources by adequate measures like community mobilization. Press and media will also have to play a major role in informing and motivating the people.

NGOs Experiences

After the enactment promulgated the country to abolish the bonded labour, some NGO's have undertaken the onerous task of freeing the child labour in carpet industry, taking into confidence the local administration including police. Raids were conducted on the premises of the carpet manufacturing factories and children shackled in servitude, were freed. At occasions, father of the child was also rescued in the raid. The children, thus freed, were sent to their homes, after the rules, according to enactment, were followed and documents prepared. An amount of Rs. 6640/- was earmarked for the parents for rehabilitation of the child. Half of the amount was paid at the time of emancipating the child and half after some period, at his home. The administration, at place of episode, paid the first instalment while the administration at his home town was to pay the second. The second one was hardly paid as it was usurped by the unscrupulous staff. The practice was distraught with a plethora of problems and bottlenecks:

- The employers resorted to Violence.
- Parents lacked the courage.
- Child was mortally afraid and traumatized, which retarded personality growth and development.
- Cooperation of administration was lukewarm.
- NGO's functionaries were threatened with dire consequences and many times actually molested or brutally and mortally beaten.
- Public cooperation was never forthcoming.

Later on, due to Supreme Court directives, the onus of paying rehabilitation cost was put upon the employer, by imposition and recovery of Rs. 20000/- as pecuniary fine. This amount was purported to be fixed and child's education and rehabilitation expenses, to be met out of the accruing interest. The provisions are flagrantly violated than actually followed. The survey conducted, as per directions of the government, in pursuance of the Supreme Court directives, proved to be a total farce as enumerators warned the employers before hand or compromised with them because of financial gains and the data published proves to be blatantly false. Therefore, how far one can except that an amount of Rs. 20000/- will be realized from the employer.

Some NGO's have opened residential schools for the freed child labour. MUKTI ASHRAM run by SACCS is one of them. The main problem, which arises, is at the time of the child having attained adulthood, he is required to leave the school and enter into mainstream of society. Financial constraints hinder adequate adjustment, which resolves into psycho-somatic manifestations going largely unattended. To take care of the child at this stage becomes of paramount importance.

Few Case Studies

We have come to know about many cases of child labour put to exploitation, violence, molestation and degradation. Attempts to emancipate them and/or rehabilitate them, have failed as the unscrupulous nexus between employer, police and administration thwart any or all the efforts of NGO's to provide help and assistance. Many a time parents relent and surrender out of fear or for pecuniary gains (paltry mostly). We will cite some case studies:

1. From an adjoining district of Lucknow, a local physician (in government services as well as having roaring private practice) bought a 10-year-old boy from the mother of a extremely poor family by paying Rs. 400/- only with golden promises to educate, feed, cloth and love the child as a family member. After the boy joined the family of the physician all promises were scattered to the wind and he was forced to back-breaking drudgery of household work from 5 a.m. to 11p.m. He was given basic survival ration with no other perks. Many a times the innocent village boy, when failed to perform a job, was mercilessly beaten. Once having broken a flowerpot, the child was beaten by iron rod and his whole body attained grievous injuries, broken bones and torn flesh. Deprived of food and water he was repeatedly beaten up, turn by turn, by each family member for a week... Apart from imprisonment, his cries or call for help were throttled. Anyhow, due to initiative of a neighbour, the case was taken up by a NGO and some

social activists. FIR was lodged in the police station. Child was rescued and court case launched against the physician. The child was medically examined and medico-legal report gave full details of the inhuman treatment meted by the child. To the frustration, anger, a sense of utter helplessness of the child, the mother of the child again compromised with the physician and back-tracked her statement. The child was again put in the servitude of the same physician and all cases have been withdrawn against him.

2. Very recently a domestic servant in a Minister's household was blamed for a theft of some money. He was imprisoned in the residence mercilessly and brutally assaulted continuously for 10 days and ultimately was thrown from 7th floor of the scraper to the ground. Evidently, all went Scot-free. The only redeeming feature was that the local public burnt the house of the minister in his hometown.

3. Shankargarh is a block of Allahabad District of Uttar Pradesh notoriously famous for bonded/child labour in silica mines. The whole family works in the mine as a unit, comprising of the father, mother and children who all help in digging, breaking stones for producing Silica sand. A network of NGO's developed their agenda for relief and rehabilitation of these labour families. Extensive surveys and public hearings were organised. Many billed the request forms for hearing. The night before the contractor and his henchmen threatened the entire area with dire consequences if anyone travelled up for hearing. A small number of victims trickled before the presiding High Court Judge and narrated their woebegone tale of blatant exploitation, abuse, shark-loaning and even women's molestation. Some specific cases are:

   - Old tottering wraith of a maternal grand mother--the only solace of two boys (11 and 8 years) took courage to present her case. Both the children were working in mines. The older one got a serious head injury from a fallen stone. The grand mother knocked the doors she could reach but no relief or rehabilitation was provided, neither by employing contractor nor by the community. The child is still in a skeletal state.

- A boy, entering the threshold of adulthood, had to get his one leg amputated because of a severe accident in the mine. At the time of hearing he was in a highly traumatized state with no prospect of any rehabilitation. All medical expenses were borne by the family. Life is in peril, if the boy narrates his tale of woes mid suffering.
- One family destined to toil in the mine has a precocious child exceptional in learning and studies. The family secretly kept him at Allahabad with some benevolent relations and he pursued his high school studies. The contractor, learning the fact, threatened to kidnap and kill the child if not brought back to work in the mine. The helpless father has no option but to obey.
- Hardly few months back a NGO functionary, after due motivation and signed permission of the parents of six children, (freed from the bondage of child labour out of stupendous zeal and courage of the worker and parents) was taking them to a rehabilitation school at Delhi for enrolments. With the connivance of local administration including police, a woman minister to win false laurels, ordered a police raid on the party. The girl functionary was attacked, beaten and locked up in spite of producing documents. Few children escaped and the rest were charged sheeted and committed to the youth correction home.
- Shankargarh silica stone mining is done by local villagers (actually tribal but denied the status by state government and listed as scheduled caste) and labour migrated from adjoining M.P. villages. The local Raja, in spite of Zamindari system abolished 50 years back, holds the rights of 80% land of the area which he leases to big contractors, who sub-let it to sub-contractors for silica mining. Contractors and sub contractors engage the labour and keep them in

bondage and servitude for generations. A family of four takes a fortnight to produces Silica sand worth a truck for which they are paid a pittance of Rs. 300/-, from which earlier advances loan interests are deducted. Then the same truck is sold for Rs. 3000/- right in Shankargarh and if brought to Ferozabed then it fetches Rs. 6000/-. The entire tale and trail of silica is splashed with the life and blood of child labour. Sexual molestation by the contractors and their henchmen is a repeated story.

- One sub-contractor of the Raja was demoniacally sex-starved and so the females of labour force, one by one, were forced to enter his "HAREM" every night. The local administration knew that people knew about it, but no one dared to object because the man has the patronage of Raja, who is swathed under the patronage of a ex-union defence minister (whose Air force helicopters, landing on the palace's roof, was a scene to behold and sight to appreciate). Helpless and hapless were the labourers to prevent the contractors sexual atrocities/ orgies. So when the turn of a 13-year-old girl hailing from a bonded family came, their community sent words to the dreaded dacoit of the area and solicited his protection. So one dark night the harem of the contractor was attacked and set a fire. He was roasted alive. The police, administration, Raja and his big patron left no stone unturned to punish the perpetrators of crime or justice but failed due to community's silence and non-cooperation.

Child Labour: Ground Realities

Given the limitations mentioned, what does the Indian scene look like?

1. The first thing, that must be said, is that although a defined, detailed and definitive relief map is not yet available, a number of snapshots of child labour can be pieced together. This is partly because there are differing

definitions of child labour, but primarily because no comprehensive national government survey has been conducted. The 1929 Royal Commission Investigation, while by no means comprehensive or exhaustive, still comes closest. Therefore the data that does exist comes substantially from case studies: some of them regional, others industry- specific, but most of them involving the same research methodology. What this involves is surveying sample groups of child labourers numbering from between 100 to 1000 subjects, and eliciting statistical information by means of interviews, invariably at the place of work - not the most neutral of sites, for objective responses.

2. Defining child labour as working children below the age of 15 which conforms with the Census and recent legislative indicators, the 1983 report established the following configurations:

   - The total child labour population was estimated at 43.79 million, which represented 26.7 per cent of children between the ages of 5 and 15.
   - Despite regional variation, most child labourers, especially if they worked in family related occupations, did not receive incomes. Here the north registered a low of 2 per cent of children earning income, the south a high of 10 per cent
   - Girls generally outnumbered boys: in the west zone by a significant margin.
   - A majority of working children in rural areas are illiterate. In urban areas, the balance was the other way round. The illiteracy rate varying according to region and the type of work involved. Over all 64 per cent of working children were illiterate.
   - At least 80 percent of child labourers came from the Scheduled Tribes and Castes, even more in the child intensive, invariably export oriented, industries like, carpet making or gemstone polishing.

3. What clearly emerges from all this are the limitations of the statistical record. In so far as core statistics exist, they are insufficient to pinpoint the exact magnitude and dimensions of child labour. Statistics that purport to 'capture' these attributes in one number only serve to disguise the complexity of the phenomenon.

Distorted and Vitiated Arguments

Poverty

In the general group, poverty is always cited first and received the most emphasis, for it appears incontestable that the persistence of child labour is connected to the prevalence of poverty. With 30 percent of the Indian population, living below the government defined poverty line, children arguably have to work. While their family cannot support them, their earning capacity may be critical to their family's survival.

As the statistics indicate—the more economically backward and drought prone area, the greater the incidence of child labour. But the issue is not that simple. For those who put the equation that, poverty is the main reason for children to enter the work force, there are just as many who turn the equation around. Thus, it is frequently propounded that child labour not only perpetrates poverty, it now also constitutes its fundamental cause. To the extent that each generation of poverty stricken children become the next generation of poverty stricken adults, they have a point.

Irrespective of its circularity, however, this argument is beside the point. Even if poverty is a major cause of child labour, it is not the only or a sufficient cause of child labour. Nor is child labour the only or a sufficient cause of poverty. Should we abolish child labour, poverty would not instantly disappear as a consequence. The nexus between child labour and poverty in short, is complex rather than linear. Neither phenomenon is the sole index of the other.

Illiteracy

According to Myron Weiner, it is the failure of the educational system in India that fuels child labour. Education simply, is not available for millions of children. Despite the constitutional undertaking, education is not compulsorily in effect even at a basic level. There are not enough school for every one to go to, nor are there sufficient trained teachers to staff those, that do exist. That is part of the problem. In much of India, public education cannot be proposed as an alternative to work.

Equally important is the utility and relevance of education, especially to families on the bread-line. If the formal education, which is accessible, does not lead to employment opportunities, schooling will not emerge as an attractive or viable option to work. With indirect cost such as books and transport, not to mention, the loss of the child's earnings education does not come free either. In this situation parents may well decide if they have a choice, that it is more sensible and certainly more remunerative for children to become breadwinners as soon as they can.

Development

There is an argument that child labour represents a stage of development which all countries pass through before full blown capitalism is reached and child labour becomes obsolete, either because of technology or loss of cost effectiveness This is certainly an argument the Indian Government has used to explain away the persistence of child labour, in the sense that as India has yet to reach such a stage it has still a lot of catching up to do. It was a rational the British Royal Commissioners of 1929 also put up in defence of child labour. But it is an argument that is wearing thin.

The transition to industrial capitalism has not eliminated child labour so much as changed its nature, even in places distorted it. With the commercialisation of agriculture a huge pool of surplus labour was created that industry has not been able to utilize. In recent years, the promotion of export industries had imparted a new impetus to child labour. Where traditionally carpet making, to take an outstanding example, was confined to Kashmir, the industry has expanded its base to eastern Uttar Pradesh to take advantage of child labour catchments in adjacent Bihar and Orissa, two of the poorest states in India. The attraction for employers is a cheap, exploitable and essentially docile work force. Development in India has so far not lessened the demand for child labourers, but substantially increased it.

Solutions

- To identify the major causes of child labour in India are one thing: it is another thing to prescribe effective cures to eliminate the practice.
- Significant rifts appear when the attempt is made to link cures to causes and to lay down the thrust of the remedial strategy: whether to alleviate child labour as an interim measure or abolish it once and for all in all out assault?
- The abolition plump could be for two main mechanism of elimination: to make education compulsory for all children up to the age of 14: to establish a minimum wage for all labour.
- Compulsory Education: it is considered, would instantly do the trick. Children would be taken out of the labour market because they had to attend school. The trouble with this prescription, however, is that it rather takes for granted the prior or accompanying emplacement of a number of crucial facilitating factors. Key among them is a revolution in thinking at all levels. Parents must be convinced that having their children educated is worthwhile. The public must be persuaded to change their attitude to caste-based discrimination: something that not even Mahatma Gandhi was able to accomplish. The political will must be present. For compulsory education to work in the way envisaged, many new schools have to be built, and recurrent expenditure on education will have to increase dramatically from its present 1.9 percent of budgetary allocation. In a deregulatory economic environment such governmental intervention and expenditure may be difficult to engineer.
- The introduction of a minimum wage would make in roads into child labour, since child labour would be deprived of its price advantage. But at what cost and to whose benefit? Wages would rise, but so would prices. More expensive labour would make life more difficult for India's business classes, without necessarily making life any easier for India's poor. With child income no longer guaranteed,

family income would likely shrink. The poor will get poorer, with the duties becoming more of a burden than a financial help.

- Whether applied separately or together, neither mechanism is capable of attacking the underlying problem of poverty. Certainly child labour would disappear, but only perhaps to be replaced by child destitution, on an even greater scale. In the short term and even beyond; poverty would hardly be touched by these measures alone.
- This is, in fact, the lesson presented by Kerala, a relatively poor state, but the most literate with a rate of almost 100 per cent and the most convinced of the need for a basic education. Held up as proof that compulsory education is the appropriate antidote for child labour, the case is by no means proven. It is true that of all the states, Kerala has long devoted most resources to education and can boast one of the lowest incidences of child labour. But it has not, thereby, become immune to child labour and it has not made much of an impact on poverty. What the example of Kerala shows is that while compulsory education can help reduce the practice, it is not enough to neutralise the demand for child labour where poverty exists.
- As for alleviation, it is doubted that this approach will make the difference either. Such as child labour has been subject to legislative protection and law enforcement, it has made no difference to date. Without a complete overhaul of the regulatory machinery including policing procedures more of the same beckons as the probable outcome, child labour will continue to flourish. The lot of child labourers may be improved, but amelioration will be tantamount to continuation.
- Going down this path, the Government has introduced a Non Formal Education (NFE) to complement the formal education, but primarily, it would seem as a palliative to make child labour more palatable: to allow children both, to work during the day and receive sonic sort of an education (at night). 'Separate and essentially unequal'

looms as the end product, with a parallel, but inferior system of education being introduced.

Summary

Whatever is attempted, it is clear there are no well-trodden shortcuts. Child labour is unlikely to disappear overnight simply because this or that lever is engaged. Since child labour impacts at a number of levels, it logically should be tackled at all these levels.

Indeed, the Indian Government, as evidenced by its 1987 National Child Labour Policy, which embodies a three-pronged strategy of eradication-legislative educative and targeted what was the outcome of this proselytising fervour and conviction law, be seen by following details.

The Government of India have ratified and accepted the provisions of the Convention of the Rights of the Child declaration made by UN on 20th Nov. 1989. Besides, it is signatory to a number of other international conventions held from time to time. This very fact makes it mandatory and obligatory upon the Government to eradicate the Child labour and rehabilitate the freed children.

So far, besides the constitutional directive principles and international guarantees this work has been done half heartedly, negligently and in a lukewarm way. So the exploitation and servitude continues unabated and 55 million children are still languishing in servitude. Honourable Supreme Court gave a historical and revolutionary ruling on a PIL laying total responsibility and accountability on the State Governments for eradication/rehabilitation of child labour. It was also directed to constitute a fund of Rs. 25000 for each freed child labour (Rs. 20000 to be paid by the employer). As a preliminary step it was required that the state government will undertake a survey jointly with trade union representatives, NGOs, social workers/ activists and journalists etc.

It is most unfortunate that the survey undertaken by the Govt functionary does not include the above mentioned person from the NGO and thus is a blatant contravention of the ruling. As an eyewash, these functionaries are going to the employers of mostly organised sector and collecting data by just asking them. Which employer will agree having employed a single child as a labourer and pay Rs., 20000/- for his honest? If one or two names somehow or other are catered in the survey list, the same are struck off after obtaining some pecuniary benefits. The social activists and NGOs pursuing this activity have made checking at Allahabad, Manikpur, Banda and many other places. The same type of pattern was found existing everywhere. Thus, it makes crystal clear that government is determined to sidetrack the issue and throttle the hopes and aspirations of the people once more, by undertaking such meaningless, neglectful, frivolous and stereotype action, which was deemed to be important and primary step for compliance of the Court's ruling.

Recommendations

What is imperative is to be very clear that in no case child labour should be regulated or given any chance to be justified by providing Non Formal Education or Nutrition, health services or any other softer solutions. This will perpetuate the child labour (servitude according to SACCS definition). The strategy should be as under:

- Complete elimination of child labour, from all types of industries or avocations, depriving a child, the chance of education and rights of childhood as laid down in CRC as:
  - Right of Survival;
  - Right of Protection;
  - Right of development;
  - Right of Participation.
- However, for those children, who have spent some time in the industry and lost their early childhood education, should be provided through special schooling and rehabilitation packages.
- The inflow of more children in any avocation, should be prevented. The parents of the children should be provided employment. Minimum wages and factory acts should be made more stringent, to prevent the exploitation of child labour.

- More researches should be done on the nature of hazardous activities employing children. Child Labour Prohibition and Regulation Act, 1986, should be amended, to prevent the employment of children. Free and compulsory education is one of the positive solutions of the problem.

11

A Strategy for Rehabilitation of Working Children in Carpet Industry in Uttar Pradesh, India

Robin Garland and David Rangpal

Project Mala Schools (Non-Formal Education)

During the last two decades, the image of the carpet industry in India has been polluted by the stigma of child labour. The slur created by the concentrated and well-organised campaign has been very damaging to the industry. I can confirm this from my personal experience when I was Chief Executive of The Scottish Heritable Trust. The lack of knowledge about the nature and scope of the abuse of children in the region, led to many erroneous conclusions, which were not based upon hard facts. Our experience since then has confirmed that although work by children was, and still is, common, CHILD LABOUR IS NOT THE PROBLEM. The problem is the lack of an alternative. The parents of children, in the carpet industry, are no different in their ambitions for their children than any other parents anywhere in the world. They will send their children to school, provided the school operates properly. Sadly, the State system for primary education in rural India leaves a lot to be desired.

All children need school for early socialization. Schools are nurseries of human nature. They are the foundation of human personality. There are broadly two categories of children. One those who can afford to go to school. They are largely based in urban areas from upper and middle socio-economic class of society. The others are from disadvantaged and improvised low caste section of the society, living in villages, which need education but cannot benefit from the primary schools in villages because these schools are non-functional or lack adequate educational environment. This is the category of children who work because they do not have an alternative to work. They are designated as "child labour." "Sheer poverty" is generally speculated to be contributing to the child labour status, but it is not the major contributing factor. According to our studies, non-functional schools in villages are the major factors contributing to child labour.

The work of Project Mala is highly focused and only deals with the children working in carpet industry in India. It is a happy story of success in dealing with the problem. Because of the high profile of the luxury goods being produced, the industry has received a high proportion of the adverse publicity on the treatment of children, but few people have tried to understand the complex nature of the industry and why it operates as it does.

There is no industry in the world, where the capital to labour ratio, is so overwhelmingly in favour of labour, as it is in the oriental hand knotted carpet industry. It is probably the single most labour intensive industry in the world. In spite of its origin, dating back as far as the 5th century BC, the methods of producing hand knotted carpets have changed little. Weaving has remained a cottage industry, with most of the households in the Mirzapur-Bhadohi districts having a loom. Weaving is a family activity in which husband, wife and children are all involved. Children either works on the family loom or looms owned by others in the neighbourhood. The relationship with loom masters, outside the bond of blood, is governed by strong community sentiment, with sense of care and concern for the good of others in the community. These are proud people who have spent most of their working life in pursuit of bare necessities of existence. In view of the poor wages, a large number of people do not now have carpet weaving as their main occupation. It is often combined with agriculture, where they weave carpets during the time they are not engaged in agricultural work.

Children were being denied education, as hardly any of the

village primary schools were functioning in the carpet-weaving belt. This inevitably led to children's idle hands being used for work purposes. Carpet weaving was taken to be a productive alternative to unproductive schooling. Although official statistics showed that 95% of the villages had a school within a radius of one kilometre, the reality was vastly different. The schools that were supposed to be in existence in official records, were hard to find and of those that could be found, lacked educational facilities. These schools were important to the basic needs of society.

However, recalcitrant bureaucracy has failed to move and the primary school education system has virtually collapsed. As a consequence, the majority of children from carpet weaving families have had to sacrifice their childhood in the work place. It was a mistaken solution to think of driving out those children from work when no alternatives are available.

Having witnessed the abuse of working children in their deprivation of schooling, we still feel strongly that it is good for the industry and the future of the community that the children learn the skill of carpet weaving at an early age, provided it is not to the exclusion of their schooling. For over ten years we have had a policy not to prevent a child from acquiring the traditional skills of their family. What we have been doing is providing an alternative to work, thereby changing the thinking and priorities of the weaving community rather than trying to impose change. We have been encouraged by the positive result. We have so far rehabilitated over 1,000 children, not including the 900 currently attending our schools, of which 300 pass out each year. We have translated the National Policy on Child Labour, 1987, into action. Our work has, however, been a drop in the ocean, due to the financial limitations of our charity. (Refer Tables 1-2)

For the last ten years, Project Mala has operated within the carpet-weaving belt, seeking out the poorest villages to offer the weaving families hope of a better life for their children by providing:

- non-formal education which is at least as good as any formal education available through the State system;
- skill training which ensures their ability to earn a living for themselves and their family;
- daily nutritional meal providing about 1100 calories, comprehensive medical care and immunization,

TABLE 1
Project Mala Enrolments in Schools 1990-2000
Mirzapur-Bhadhoi Carpet Weaving Belt (Uttar Pradesh)

Name of Centre	*Carried Forward*	*New Enrollments*	*Dropouts*	*Passed out*
Guria	1193	774	78	439
Hasra	493	385	66	169
Amohi	490	419	39	230
Pathera	486	405	46	209
Mujhera	198	152	2	—
All Mala Schools	2760	2135	231	1047

TABLE 2
Project Mala Schools
Budget Revenue for the Financial Year 1999-2000

Budget Head	*Expenditure (1999-2000)*						
	Administration	*Guria*	*Majhera*	*Hasra*	*Pathera*	*Amoi*	*Total*
Teachers and staff Salary	377,400	185,400	127,800	127,800	127,800	127,600	1,074,000
Health Care		16,500	8,250	8,250	8,250	8,250	49,500
Nutrition		421,200	210,600	210,600	210,600	210,600	1,263,600
Extra Curricular		3,600	1,800	1,800	1,800	1,800	10,800
Teaching Aids		92,000	58,000	58,000	58,000	58,000	324,000
School Uniform		42,000	21,000	21,000	21,000	21,000	126,000
Examination		5,200	2,600	2,600	2,600	2,600	15,600
Building/Equip	15,000	7,200	3,600	3,600	3,600	3,600	36,600
Rehabilitation		200,000	—	100,000	100,000	100,000	500,000
Recruitment	12,000	—	—	—	—	—	12,000
Printing and Sta.	13,000	—	—	—	—	—	13,000
Travel	60,000	—	—	—	—	—	60,000
Rentals	43,600	—	—	—	—	—	43,600
Post and Telcom	50,000	—	—	—	—	—	50,000
Motor Expenses	85,000	—	—	—	—	—	85,000
Audit Etc;	35,000	—	—	—	—	—	35,000
Meeting	30,000	—	—	—	—	—	30,000
Contingencies	36,050	48,655	21,683	26,683	26,683	26,683	186,435
Overheads	757,050	252,350	126,175	126,175	126,175	126,175	—
Total Running Cost	1,514,000	1,274,105	581,508	686,508	686,508	686,508	3,915,135
No. of Children		300	150	150	150	150	900
Cost per Child (Rs.)		4,247	3,877	4,577	4,577	4,577	4,350

Source: Deputy Chairman and Executive Officer, Project Mala.

- management of specific health problems and routine ailments and nutritional deficiency.

A variety of extra curricular activities include instruction in personal hygiene and development of the right attitude towards work, which will help them in negotiating their rights from a position of strength. We also help them in their rehabilitation on completion of three years schooling

The Project

Project Mala has developed as a system strategy for rehabilitation of working children in the Carpet Industry with Non-formal and Vocational Education as its vehicle. It has been based on four firm assumptions, derived from the studies in the child labour situation in the districts of Varanasi and Mirzapur.

One, that carpet weaving is a productive alternative to unproductive schooling, suggesting that village schools are non-functional and children have no business to be there. The functional poverty of village schools is so amply documented that few challenge the accuracy of such reports.[1]

Two, the problem of working children in carpet industry is basically their abuse. This abuse is deprivation of childhood rights--education, health-care, nutrition and recreation. These are the growth factors in a child's personality. Childhood, deprived of these growth factors is a lost childhood. A lost childhood cannot be compensated, but could be regained by quick intervention of education. Whilst, formal education protects childhood from being lost, the non-formal facilitates its restoration. Both are supportive to any system strategy for protection and rehabilitation of working children.

Three, that payment of stipend as envisaged in the National Child Labour Projects (NCLP) was a mistaken kindness. In the beginning we paid stipend of Rs.100 for each child in our schools on accumulated basis by cheque. The thinking behind this scheme was that it would facilitate rehabilitation of children passing out, on the conclusion of 3 years of schooling. From the very beginning, we were not in favour of giving stipend to compensate families, for the loss of income, they speculatively experienced in sending their working children to school, because there was no such loss noted in our maiden survey for identification and enrolment. The children earning around Rs.100 were not to come to school. This was nine years back. They were in age group 12+. The willing seekers of school enrolment included children in age group 9+, working on family loom or engaged in work preparatory to weaving or who were potential child labour. We preferred the 10+ age group for 3-year schooling, for the simple reason that by the time they complete schooling; they would attain adulthood to escape possible exploitation as child labour. An accumulated stipend @ Rs. 100 per month over a period of three years was considered good for regular attendance and for rehabilitation support on passing out. Studies on how this was used for the children passed out of our school in year 1993 and 1994 revealed that it was used for rehabilitation of a microscopic minority of children. In majority of cases, it was spent on dowries, general household expenses or even the repayment of loans. This scheme was, therefore, changed into a Rehabilitation Plan, but having implemented it for two years we found that rehabilitation benefits were also not used for children and parents involved themselves in breach of trust. '*Rehabilitation*' as it used to be called was withdrawn, effective from April 2000, leaving only the continuation of our Advance Weaving Academy to rehabilitate ex-Mala students for training in advance weaving skills. Withdrawal of stipendiary benefits has not cut down the enrolment. Instead, children have queued for enrolment for the academic session beginning July 1999. An opinion survey revealed that it was the Mala schools which were in demand and not the stipend.

Four, that as a consequence of above, a large number of parents showed themselves no different in their ambition for their children than any other parents anywhere in the world and were found in the queue with even their earning children in age group 11+. This proved our strategy for rehabilitation of working children positive. Coming back to the alternative to work i.e. education, Project Mala System Strategy for protection of children from "abuse" by world's single most labour intensive industry and their instant employment, has been greatly facilitated by non-formalizing the State Primary Education for the following reasons.

- To reinstate Primary Education System, which has gone down to an Examination System for Pass Certificate are both farce.
- To restructure and diversify State Primary Education courses of study, by condensation of formal education text materials, making it need based and manageable within

the NFE time frame.

- To combine science and social studies into one subject of Environment Study, for use of *Evs* texts for development of skills in reading and writing Hindi language in the process of making children aware of their environment - every things that surround them and affect their social lives.
- To make teaching and learning process, activity-based, for accelerated pace of learning necessary for disadvantaged and slow learners.
- To monitor Minimum Level of Learning (MLL) by continuous internal assessment of learners and remedial teaching.
- To combine NFE with Vocational Education to make it work based for instant rehabilitation of the majority of children in the carpet industry, on the conclusion of their 3 year schooling, leaving only few bright ones for collegiate education.
- To experiment Gandhian approach to basic education in rural India for its relevance in the changed social time and space
- To make school supervision intensive for monitoring all-important spheres of school life, particularly for on-the-spot in service teachers' education, demanding that school programme is fully understood, appreciated and practised by them.

The only problem, NGOs have faced, is in authentication of the pass certificates of Class V children for mainstreaming them into the post primary stage of formal system of education in State Middle Schools. There has not been clear policy statement for the same from the State Education Directorate, and moreover the District Education authorities have been non-cooperative and demanding. It has tested our patience.

Project Mala Schools

Project Mala was started in January 1990, with a single school in the village of Guria in the Varanasi district. It now has five schools extending out into the tribal areas in the Mirzapur district. The curriculum is need based, assuring basic literacy, numeracy and general knowledge of environment in conformity with the standards laid down in the State primary school syllabus. In addition, children receive vocational skills to best equip them in life in these remote parts of the country.

Project Mala has been a spectacular success. Not only have the children in our schools responded well to non-formal and vocational education, but also after three years they have been academically equal to the children attending State schools. So far, all of the children who have taken State primary education examination at Grade V have passed and of those, over 50% have gone to join the State secondary education system.

The health care component has been equally successful. Children have come to our schools suffering from a variety of health problems. Malnutrition, polio, scabies and worms have been common in new children. The School Physician has given all new children a thorough medical examination and further health checks have been carried out in each term. The children have been given a balanced nutritional mid-day meal each day to a level of eleven hundred calories. After a year at the school, most of their health problems have been overcome and the children show a distinct clinical improvement.

As can be seen from our annual budget, the total cost of running Project Mala, including all student supplies, vocational training, health care programme, nutrition, rehabilitation and administration costs is less than Rs. 40,00,000 per year for 900 children. This works out at just over Rs. 4,000 per child per year. This figure has been reduced over the years, partly as a result of favourable exchange rates, but mostly through economies made within the project. As an example, we now grow almost 10% of our own food. Project Mala is innovative in style and experimental in character. An ongoing study of our work has highlighted two main areas of new development:

1. a need to extend the area of geographical coverage to combat abusive child labour in specific areas;
2. a need to provide advanced training in carpet weaving, to the students passing out of our schools, to facilitate their rehabilitation and to modernise weaving technology for the enhancement of weaving efficiency.

The geographical development should be combined with a closer working relationship with other NGOs. It is sad for us that the development of new schools is such a disjointed affair with State and NGOs working in the same area but never talking to one another. Part of the problem is that we are all in competition for the same finance. This has led to a piecemeal approach to the placement of schools and school sites being chosen by location rather than need.

Whilst there have been a number of new schools introduced, there is no co-ordination to provide uniform standards and no infrastructure to guarantee a sustainable financial or administrative future.

We in Project Mala believe that the correct approach would be to take a whole block of a district and deal with it on a permanent basis. By dealing with a whole block we would be able to make a detailed survey of the area and strategically place schools to ensure minimum walking distances for the children and the right size to cope with future needs. Linking new schools with an administrative set-up, capable of being ultimately self-sustaining by the local community, is an important part of our thinking. We believe that the local communities are the best people to run their own schools as they have the interest and the ability to do so. We have already, to some extent, proved this by our policy of developing local people as teachers for our schools. It was no surprise to us that in the annual assessment of our schools and subsequent performances, the school located in the remote villages and tribal areas won our internal prize for the best school.

We in Project Mala have strongly felt that it will be a mistaken kindness to chase the children from loom without providing an alternative i.e. properly functional schools. Without these schools to go, chasing could have been worst than child labour. Project Mala experiment in non-formalization of State Primary Education System has been a success. Prof. C.J. Daswani, the then Head of the Department of NFE, NCERT found our NFE model as worth adoption, across the country, for working children and advocated it on all platforms. Dr. (Mrs) P. Das Gupta of the Department, who made an assessment of our educational programme has seen it as a unique innovation in NFE for personal growth and professional development of working children and their rehabilitation on the conclusion of 3 years schooling. A recent Study of Schools of NGOs for working children in carpet industry in the Mirzapur and Bhadohi districts conducted by Dr. Zutshi, has ranked Project Mala schools on the top on all performance levels. The Working Group on Contemporary Forms of Slavery received a presentation of Project Mala System

Strategy for Rehabilitation of Working Children in Carpet Industry, to the United Nations with appreciation in its twenty-fourth Session (28-31 June 1999) at Geneva.

Reference

1. Citizen's Initiative on Elementary Education in India published by the Core Group C.J. Daswani, Sanjoy Ghosh and J. Acharya, on Teachers Day, September 5,1997

12

An Overview of International Programme on Elimination of Child Labour (IPEC) Programmes in India

R.K. Khurana

Introduction

From its very inception in 1919, the International Labour Organization (ILO) has been concerned about the employment of children. This concern has been reflected in the series of Conventions and Recommendations adopted by the ILO from 1919 onwards. Convention No. 5, "Fixing the Minimum Age for Admission of Children to Industrial Employment," is the first of them and the other important are Convention No. 138 and Convention No. 182 concerning "Minimum Age for Admission to Employment" (1973), with its accompanying Recommendation No. 146 and "Elimination of Worst Forms of Child Labour" respectively. These Conventions and Recommendations have helped to establish standards for the employment of children worldwide.

The task of assisting member states to be able to apply these standards nationally and ratify the conventions has also moved apace in the ILO. Most important amongst recent initiatives in ILO's technical co-operation activities on child labour, has been the

International Programme on the Elimination of Child Labour (IPEC). IPEC is a global initiative of the ILO launched in 1992 to support participating member countries in their national efforts to combat and eliminate child labour progressively, while simultaneously creating a world wide movement against it. The ILO-IPEC programme is flexible in responding to the country's needs in addressing their specific child labour situation.

India was the first country to sign a Memorandum of Understanding (MOU) with the ILO for implementing IPEC, and is currently targeting the highest number of children under the programme anywhere in the world. The MOU, signed in 1992, laid down the principles, areas and modalities of cooperation between the Indian Government and the ILO for the elimination of child labour. It was agreed that the cooperation would be based on ILO Conventions, in particular, Convention No. 138, with the aim of *progressively eliminating* child labour and increasing awareness of its adverse effects, with solutions for its reduction and elimination.

The terms of cooperation, as outlined in the MOU, are such that the programme would be implemented through various Action Programmes, selected by a National Steering Committee of the Ministry of Labour. This committee includes representatives of the Government, representatives of employers' and workers' organizations and representatives of NG0s active in the field of child labour. The Secretary of the Ministry of Labour is its chairperson.

A total of 99 agreements have been signed for implementing Action Programmes under IPEC in India. Of these, 57 were funded using the US$ 2.251 million allotted to India in the 1992-93 biennial budget of IPEC. Forty-two Action Programmes have been funded from the US$ 1.4 million allotted to India in the 1994-95 biennial budget. Of the 57 agreements signed in 1992-93, in all but two cases, the Action Programmes have been completed. Of those signed in 1994-95, many continued into 1996.

Most of the Action Programmes of 1992-93 were implemented through NGOs. The programmes provided education in part-time or full-time, non-formal education centres. This was envisaged as a prelude to enrollment into schools. They were all designed to illustrate to the local communities that child labour is not inevitable. Over 29,000 child labourers were covered in these Action Programmes. To increase the institutional capacity of NG0s implementing IPEC projects on child labour, three training programmes were held. The programmes focussed on improving the management, evaluation and design of Action Programmes on child labour, using materials developed within IPEC.

Between the 1994-95, IPEC attracted many new partners and began working with trade unions (INTUC, BMS, CITU) and employers' organizations. It also joined hands with institutions like the Central Board for Workers Education (CBWE) and the National Safety Council (NSC). The former was a project to introduce modules on child labour into the Board's on-going workers' education programmes and the latter sought to raise the safety and health awareness of child labourers, their parents and the community. The economic aspects of child labour received attention in 1994-95 through an examination of the feasibility of replacing children with adults, in a few selected industries.

While direct support for child labourers continued in 1994-95, the emphasis shifted from merely providing welfare inputs to looking at a host of other possible strategies that could lead to a sustained action for the progressive elimination of child labour. Thus, the Action Programmes attempted to link with the local educational system, with youth groups and with women's groups.

Thirty-Six mini programmes were also funded, for less than US $ 2000 each, by IPEC during the 1994-95 biennium. These included workshops on child labour, the preparation of reports and documents, and so on.

At the national level, while the Government of India has been concerned with child labour ever since the country's independence in 1947, the 1980s saw mused initiatives against child labour, catalysed by government efforts. These included the promulgation of a new law on child labour called the Child Labour (prohibition and regulation) Act, which entered the statute books in 1986, and the framing of a National Child Labour Policy in 1987. The entry of the Government of India into ILO's, IPEC programme in 1992 indicated the government's growing concern about child labour and the need to act against it. The advent of IPEC in India coincided with government initiatives to tackle the problem systematically. These included the historic declaration made on 15 August 1994, India's Independence Day, by the then Prime Minister Shri P. V. Narasirnha Rao. The government resolved to end child labour in hazardous industries by 2000 A.D, and set up of a special fund of Rs. 850 crores (US$ 250 million) for this purpose. A National Authority for the

Elimination of Child Labour was established to oversee the implementation of schemes using the fund.

The Ministry of Labour, Government of India in addition to its own funds received financial support, under the International Labour Organization – International Programme for Elimination of Child Labour (ILO-IPEC) and under the Child Labour Action Support Programme (CLASP) aided by Government of Germany, for the operation of NCLP scheme in the identified areas. A sum of US $ 6.9 million or 270 million rupees under ILO-IPEC scheme was provided to central employees' organizations, central trade union organizations and NGOs between 1992-1999 for opening NFE schools under the NCLP.[1] Firstly, this amount has been utilized under 160 projects benefiting about 100,000 children[2] and secondly the scheme is extended till 21.12.2001 and is extendable by a further period of one year.

An Assessment of the IPEC Programme in India

The progress that IPEC made during its two phases and the challenges faced today, are explained under the following two headings: (a) The achievements, effectiveness and strengths of the IPEC Programme; and (b) the weaknesses of the programme.

Achievements, Effectiveness and Strengths of the IPEC Programme

- The IPEC approach was extremely flexible and offered the partner organizations ample scope for determining independently the level and type of intervention required. Each project could thus be developed for the specific area or situation at hand. The ability to develop strategies on an experimental basis helped foster new approaches.
- The direct funding of implementing agencies by the ILO was its strength. It saved the implementing agencies time and energy by reducing the bureaucratic problems generally associated with projects in which the funding is routed through government departments.
- Another strength of these programmes was that they brought together a large number of NG0s working on child labour, enabling them to coordinate and share experiences. The diversity of NG0s and geographical areas covered

has fostered a good beginning and established a more concrete basis for future work.

- Another significant achievement has been the ability of IPEC to show that children can be weaned away from work into schools, substituting work with education. The educational initiatives have already begun to show results. The overwhelming response to non-formal education, as well as enrollment into regular schools, shows that education plays a vital role in the process of reducing child labour.
- IPEC played a major role in involving trade unions and employer's organizations in combating child labour. Trade unions and employer's organizations have been sensitised and they have taken up the task enthusiastically. They have come up with several new initiatives. IPEC anticipates their greater involvement in future programmes.
- Organizations, such as the National Institute of Rural Development, the National Safety Council, the Central Board for Workers Education and the State Labour Institutes have been introduced to the issues of child labour and involved in the movement against it. Institutes are capable of sustaining the momentum against child labour even after IPEC ends.
- Many strategies for the elimination of child labour have been developed and can be replicated.
- This has been by far the most crucial intervention of the programme and the most effective. The main thrust, of this element of the programme, was to increase the awareness and understanding of a wide section of society about child labour. Thus, the target groups ranged from working children, their parents and employers to teachers, community and religious leaders, enforcement officers and government officials. The increased attention that child labour is now receiving as an issue of public concern can, to some extent, be attributed to IPEC's efforts.
- Contrary to the belief at the beginning of the programme, the response from working children, their parents and the community at large, to education as an alternative to work, has been overwhelming. Initial successes at rehabilitation, visibly demonstrating the advantages of education,

convinced parents to send their children to schools. Even the loss of income did not diminish the acceptance of education as a viable alternative. It must be noted, however, that the success of the rehabilitation projects owes a great (deal to the emphasis on mainstreaming children into formal schools in the later projects. Difficulties in obtaining admission, procuring uniforms and books, and lack of academic assistance at home, are strong deterrents for children wishing to go to school and contribute to the drop-out rate. Once these problems are addressed, children are more willing to enrol in regular schools).

Weaknesses of IPEC

- While recognizing these strengths, several weaknesses in the IPEC programmes can also be pointed out. They are largely managerial or administrative shortcomings in the Direct Support Action Programmes.
- There is no structured procedure for selecting projects and/or NGOs.' As a result, IPEC found itself dealing with a large number of diverse NG0s. Lack of comprehensive information on NGOs and the work being done in the field, coupled with the urgency to get the programme off the ground, resulted in IPEC's unstructured character from the beginning.
- While flexibility had certain advantages, the other side of the coin was that expectations were often not clear. The implementing agency found itself, in several instances, unable to gauge the level of impact expected and unclear about the design of the programme and the system of reporting.
- Both the implementing agencies and ILO felt that the contractual period, which was in most cases a maximum of eighteen months, was too short to register an impact. For the task at hand a longer time frame was needed for each programme.
- This situation was aggravated by the fact that the ILO-IPEC office was highly understaffed. Dealing with a very large number of projects all over the country, in an environment in which telephones, trains and communication systems are often unreliable, required a larger coordinating team.

- Many of the partner organizations found the IPEC system of reporting very elaborate and unnecessarily complex. As a result, little meaningful.
- Although guidelines exist for determining eligibility of NGOs to be considered, as well as for programmes to be selected yet. This process generated too much paper work and provided insufficient information.
- Although a large number of NG0s were brought together under this programme, the interaction between them, was limited. While it would have helped to share experiences and learn from them, there were few opportunities to do so.
- There was insufficient monitoring and evaluation of the projects in the field. This was to some extent, a function of the lack of personnel at ILO, which made it impossible for the coordinator to make frequent visits to all the projects. Lack of regional offices or regional coordinators, who could have provided periodic reports from their regions, made monitoring of projects a very difficult task. With the exception of Mini Programmes to evaluate Action Programmes, there was no other evaluation by ILO-APEC. This, coupled with the fact that the implementing agencies were unable to provide sufficient information in their reports, translated into poor documentation from the field. While a great deal of good work was done, it was largely un-documented. For example, there were many Direct Support Programmes that provided non-formal education along with vocational skills, however, their reports do not elaborate on what sort of teaching was provided, or what vocational skills were taught. Questions arise; such as, does the programme include literacy, are the vocational skills marketable, is there a sufficient demand for the products of those skills. Without this information little can be learned for future project design. Similarly, specific information on the level of participation of the working children, their parents or the communities was not well documented.
- Another weakness in the programmes, beginning with the proposals themselves, was the lack of socio-economic background information about the target groups. Generally

the projects did not furnish information on variables such as age, ethnicity, family income, etc. Such information could provide important insights into the genesis of the problem and therefore be useful in evolving a solution. Conducting baseline surveys would also be a useful exercise.

- There is now a lot of debate on this issue, particularly from the experiences of income generating projects for women, those skills like basket-weaving, pickle-making and other such traditional skills do not generate sufficient income. Where do the women take the baskets/pickles? Who do they sell them to? What is the demand for baskets or pickles? Even the gender-wise distribution is rarely provided, except in a handful of cases.

REFERENCES

1. Dr. L. Mishra, (2000) 'Child Labour in India, Problems, Constraints and Challenges,' paper presented in Trade Union Workshop, July 14-16,
2. *Ibid*.

13

Reha Programmes and Issues on the Rehabilitation of the Carpet Children

Geeta Singh

We all know that the work of NGOs, in the carpet industry of India, for eradicating child labour, has already acquired a status of model in the context of overall movement against child labour in India and abroad. This was mainly due to the overall impact created on the existing child labour situation in the industry. The campaign against child labour in the carpet industry has been considered as successful because it resulted in involving several agencies—both governmental and non-governmental, national and international, bilateral and multilateral agencies for the cause of child labour and establishing ethical practices in carpet manufacturing. Several agencies also took work of rehabilitating child labourers related to the carpet industry. These agencies have achieved considerable success in the eradication and rehabilitation of child labourers from the industry. The Reha Programme is one of the major initiatives taken in this field.

Background—Reha Programme

Reha Programme supports and seeks to rehabilitate working,

freed or potential child labourers related to carpet industry of India. The plight of thousands of children working in the carpet industry received focused attention with the heightened activity of *'carpet campaign'* launched by some national and international NGOs from the year 1990 onwards. Among these NGOs, SACCS (South Asian Coalition on Child Servitude), played a major role in the release of children through its raid and rescue operations in the carpet industry. Subsequently, a strong *'consumer awareness'* campaign launched by it in Europe and North America was hailed by several international groups, trade unions and donor agencies from Europe and other parts of the world. Perhaps, this was a unique partnership between southern and northern NGO's, which actively collaborated to fight for the total eradication of child labour working in the carpet industry of India. Among these international agencies some of them were funding agencies that were actively participating in the 'consumer campaign' in their respective countries. Thus, the partnership between Indian NGOs and these agencies were not the usual funders implementers relationship but an interactive 'action-oriented' relationship. The carpet *"consumer campaign"* had its effect felt in several quarters including governments, importer organisations, trade promotion councils etc. At that time, the American Senate was also considering a bill, called as *"Tom Harkins Bill"*, to boycott all such products, which were made by the use of child labour. Thus, there was a possibility of Indian carpet getting boycotted by the consumers of the importing countries. To save the industry from this eventuality, the partners of carpet campaign initiated the formation of a licenser company *"Rugmark Foundation"* which was indeed a remarkable initiative to promote product ethical practices in the competitive phase of globalisation. After this initiative, several developments followed, resulting in the creation of social and administrative pressure on the employer of the children, for releasing them from work. These developments, which led to the release of thousands of children, further created apprehension of many more children being released. But, the administration was not prepared to rehabilitate them. Hence, there was a possibility of these children going back to work. It was at this juncture that some of the carpet campaign partners came together and initiated *Reha Programme* in 1994 with noble intentions of rehabilitating these children.

Vision and Objectives

Vision statement of Reha Programme reads as follows:

"Development of the child in community, with a focus on children, in relation to carpet industry, whereby they are enabled to enjoy human rights and exercise social duties towards the formation of a just world order based on values such as equality, sharing cooperation and common good".

Guided by the above vision, the main thrust of Reha Programmes is preventing potential child labourers from entering into the labour force and rehabilitation of freed working children. All the Reha supported Programmes are based on the following fundamental premise:

- Child labour is essentially not a "*harsh reality*" but is a part of "*distorted reality*" created and supported by vested interest groups for their own benefit.
- All children have similar potential growth, irrespective of their socio-economic background, provided they are given the required developmental avenues.

The Reha Programmes strives to achieve the following objectives:

- Demonstrating through its work the possibilities of development in ex-child labourers and deprived children by providing them opportunities and means of development.

- Influencing the policies of government and multilateral agencies to change their policies in favour of deprived children and creating pressure on the concerned authorities for effective implementation of existing provisions.

The organisational structure of Reha Programmes:

The donor agencies namely Bread for the world (Bfw), Misereor, Terre des hommes (Tdh) of Germany and Christian Aid from UK formed *Reha Consortium* to pool in their resources under the

Reha Fund for supporting this programme of the carpet children. The Indian Reha Committee (IRC) is an intermediary body which is constituted for the purpose of selecting quality Reha Projects and recommending the same for sanction to GRC, formulating policies related to this programme, training, supervising and providing technical support to the Reha project partners. This committee is constituted of representatives from NGOs who were involved in carpet campaign, representatives of funding agencies and independent experts on education and rehabilitation. The Indian Reha Secretariat (IRS) was setup to primarily execute all the functions of IRC. It is responsible for organising various kinds of training programme for its project partners and providing them other technical support. The Reha Secretariat also conducts feasibility study of projects along with their monitoring and evaluation. It functions as a link between project implementer, the Indian Reha Committee and the Reha Consortium.

Current Major Activities undertaken under the Reha Programmes

Promotional Activities

We have been doing promotional activities to extend the reach of the programme to the far-flung areas and unattended population. In this, we identify NGOs active in remote target areas and provide the required training and orientation for participating in the programme.

Identification of New Command and Catchment Areas

A constant attention is also paid on identifying new areas where still there is less social intervention or where new carpet manufacturing units are being setup. For example, we are now paying attention to Madhubani district of Bihar, Sonbhadra of U.P. and the carpet belt of Rajasthan.

Training and Orientation Programme on Cooperatives:

An important concern of Reha Programmes is to assist in employment generation and income augmentation of source group. It is found that, particularly in the labour catchment area of carpet industry, there is very less potential of employment. In such a case, the children passing out of NFE's may again find themselves without options. Thus, the Secretariat is currently focusing on the promotion of group enterprises i.e. cooperatives, self help group, women thrift groups, etc. From these activities it is expected that the children coming out of the rehabilitation centres and their families can get employment opportunities and would increase collective efforts among members of focus groups.

Recently, the Reha Secretariat has facilitated an orientation field visit for a project partner to some of the successful cooperatives of Karim Nagar and Warrangal districts of Andhra Pradesh. These visits have encouraged the project partners to speed up the process of formation of cooperatives in Palamau district of Bihar.

Capacity Building and Training Programmes

One of the regular activities of Reha Programme is to organise training programme for its partners and potential partners according to their need. We are preparing, training programmes for perspective development of NGOs, on rehabilitation. These training programmes would also assist potential partners in technical aspects like project designing, developing concepts on planning, monitoring and evaluation.

Impact and Achievements

As stated earlier, Reha Programme was started in 1994 for rehabilitation of children in the carpet industry. It has distinction of working in both command and catchment areas of the carpet industry. Out of the 13 projects supported by Reha since 1994-98, six were running in the command area of U.P. (Mirzapur, Bhadohi, Sonbhadra, Gazipur and Banda) and four were running in the catchment areas of Bihar in the districts of Saharsa, Patna and Samastipur along with another project on campaign and awareness with regard to rehabilitation in both U.P. and Bihar. Besides this, there were two research projects undertaken on the feasibility study of cooperativisation and the study on the assessment of rehabilitation programme conducted by Dr. Zutshi.[1]

Presently, we have five projects running in Bihar and U.P. Generally these projects have the following main components.

- Providing educational facilities and vocational training

in form of NFE to children.

- Awareness generation and social mobilisation on the issue.
- Capacity building of NGOs and people's organisation to fulfill the task of rehabilitation and positive prevention.
- Income augmentation and employment generation for families of child labourers.

All these components are synergically combined. Thus, they exercise influence over each other. However, as the focus of this workshop is mainly to assess the impact of non-formal educational programme run by various agencies, I would like to restrict myself, to the ways and means of strengthening the efficacy of NFE's, which is the main visible component of rehabilitation programme. Till now, Reha has supported 75 NFE centres with a planned capacity of 50 children each. However, the actual numbers of the children attending these centres were much higher than the number of their planned capacity. These NFEs were different from each other in respect of their location, school timings, syllabus and quality of manpower. Thus, due to their heterogeneity, it is rather difficult to give a concrete assessment of their impact. However, the fact that these centres were attended by numbers nearly twice of their planned capacity, indicates their significance and need.

Following are some of the general impacts of the Reha Programme based on the field observations and secondary sources (some of these have also been reflected in Dr. Zutshi's assessment report).

1. Creating Opportunities for Development

The NFE provided first ever access to basic education, vocational training and health care to the children related to the carpet industry (working, freed, potential). Most of these children were the first generation of learners in their families. Simultaneously, it also created multiple entry points to formal schools for these deprived children. A sizeable percentage of these children after completion of NFE have joined formal schools.

2. Awareness in the Community

These NFEs created a kind of cultural shock in the 'Source Communities'. For many of these communities these NFEs were the first social intervention of any kind. It created awareness regarding ill effects of child labour and prepared a ground for communities demanding their right to education. This is reflected by the participation of source communities and ex-child labourers in sufficient numbers in the various rallies and protest marches organised by the implementing agencies.

3. Conducive Classrooms

In formal schools, due to prevalence of discrimination practiced on the basis of caste and class, the children of deprived communities feel disinterested in studies resulting in non-enrollment and dropout. It has been observed that in a number of schools, where teachers were selected from the same community and the local area, helped in the removal of caste and class bias from the classroom making them more conducive for learning. As an example, we can cite the work of a Reha project partner who has immensely helped the local administration in establishing NCLP (National Child Labour Project) schools in the Saharsa district of Bihar. The location and selection of teachers was mainly done by this NGO, which took special care in selecting teachers from the same caste as that of the focus group. In this case, it was the mushar caste. The result was that the performance of NCLP schools of Saharsa was the best in Bihar.

4. Bringing Change in Schooling Culture

The NFE centres have also cultivated a new kind of relationship, marked with a more cordial and friendly learning atmosphere between the teachers and students. These centres, which are also characterised by the joyful nature of education, make way for friendly and interested teachers instead of following the old authoritarian tradition of teaching. Hence, this culture of non-formal education can be later induced in the formal system to make it more interesting for the children.

5. Reduction in Employment of Children

There has been a decline, in the number of children employed in the carpet industry, at an early age, due to increased awareness, in source community and other sections of society, on the existing legal provisions and ill effects of employing children. The NFE's also provided a positive alternative to the working children and potential child labourers, reducing possibilities of their employment.

According to Dr. Zutshi's report only 8.62% child labourers were found in looms currently operating in the villages with NFE schools.

6. *Positive Prevention*

These NFEs provided an alternative to potential child labourers thus preventing them to join the labour force. In Reha schools there was a good percentage of 'nowhere children', which signifies the need of permanent alternative to reduce the chances of potential child labourers joining work.

7. *Increased Participation of Civil Society Organisations*

Earlier, there were several non-governmental organisations including Human Right Groups, Trade Unions, Voluntary Agencies etc., which were neutral with respect to the issue on eradication of child labour from the carpet industry. However, due to the initiative taken by the Reha Programme for rehabilitating these children and the positive results emerging from it, many of these organisations became active regarding this issue resulting in more intensive non-governmental activities in the carpet belt. Several other agencies, both governmental and international, started supporting the initiative of the NGOs by providing them with required resources.

The above mentioned reflects the main effects of Reha Programmes. These points should be considered in relation to Dr. Zutshi's report.

Suggestions and Remarks

Although rehabilitation programmes are still in their nascent stage, the present study has given us a chance to collectively reflect over the various on-going rehabilitation programmes.

It appears that the movement against child labour has evolved in a lop-sided manner in which the maximum emphasis was on the policy intervention for eradication of child labour but not much thought about alternatives. Perhaps this may be the only way in which social movements are developed. It is because of this reason that the form and structure of rehabilitation programme has not been very clear. Nevertheless, with the issue of rehabilitation gaining prominence, the search for alternatives has become inevitable.

Through experiences in Reha and other agencies, involved in the rehabilitation of child labourers related to the carpet industry, it has been established beyond doubt that the role of NFE is indispensable till infrastructure of formal schooling and quality schooling is available to each child of this country.

Lots of work has been done to improve the quality of education in formal schools but not much has been done to provide quality education to the deprived children. The former (formal schools) are comparatively easier to undertake, as the children are already in the schools, but in the latter case, most of the children are the first generation learners without any external support for fulfilling their need of education. Thus, the field of non-formal education and rehabilitation has become more challenging.

Although it is true that NFEs were initiated to fulfill the requirement of formal schools and to suit the diverse life style of rural India, nevertheless, they should still have their indigenous characteristic fully in resonance with the local life style and aspirations. Unfortunately, the existing NFEs are generally poor substitutes of formal schools. Thus, the present form of NFEs is not very effective and useful. The prescriptive nature of NFE planning should pave way for more decentralised and locally meaningful plans.

Following are suggestions, which have emerged from field observations and reflection of my colleagues involved in the work:

A. Similarity in Form and Structure of NFE Centres:

Variety in approaches is considered as one of the important characteristics of NFE's, since it can suit varying target groups located in different social and geographical location. Nevertheless, NFE should not be treated as 'formless'. Some basic parameters should be decided for constructing NFE programme. For example, hours of teaching should be same in all schools, though timings can be varied. These parameters would enhance the homogeneity in structure and function of NFE's that in turn will facilitate the monitoring and evaluation of the programme, a set of parameters can be developed for schools sponsored by a particular funding agency or Consortium.

B. Linkage with Panchayati Raj Institution

After the 73rd constitutional amendment and enactment of the Panchayati Raj legislation, the Panchayati Raj Institutions (PRI) has got some authority in respect of development and education.

Till date, not much has been done in this direction. Some kind of initiative could also make programme sustainable, since some resources are now available at Panchayat level. But these linkages need to be developed carefully so that feudal tendencies existing in these institutions may not mar its natural growth.

C. Linkage with projects like DPEP

The possibility of linking up NFE programme with projects like DPEP (District Primary Education Projects) and other such similar governmental and non-governmental projects, which have also the policy of decentralised planning, should be sought wherever possible.

D. Teachers Training: Interlinkages with the governmental institutions

The teachers training are the key ingredients of any educational programme. The NGOs entrusted with the task of running NFEs do not have adequate infrastructure for providing quality training to their teachers. On the other hand, there is a vast network of teachers training institute under central and state governments, as the government has the constitutional obligation of providing education to all children below 14 years of age. Besides this, the *National Policy on Education 1986*, further confirms the government stand to support NFE and ensure its education quality to be at par with formal schools. Thus, there is sufficient ground for developing collaboration with governmental organisations for periodic teachers training to improve the quality of education in NFEs. These trained teachers can later be utilised by the government in the process of universalisation of elementary education.

E. Monitoring and Crisis Management System

For successful implementation of rehabilitation projects, it is essential to monitor the projects periodically and consistently. The donor and intermediary agencies should evolve a monitoring and crisis management system to ensure unobstructed and effective implementation of the project. This unit can work in coordination with local village committee or other such people's committee.

F. Mass Mobilisation and Pressure Building

The project implementing agencies should try to mobilise local mass support during the project implementation period and should start building pressure on local and district level governmental authorities to take over the NFE. This demand would be in consonance with the *National Policy on Education 1986*, which states that in absence of formal schooling facilities, the concerned government should provide non-formal education where quality will be equivalent to that of formal schools.

G. Emphasis on Comprehension of Locally Meaningful Subjects

Though in principle, it has already been accepted, by the concerned educationist and agencies, that education should be based on learners need and should be related to the local environment. Unfortunately, in practice not much has been achieved in this respect. This is also substantiated in Dr. Zutshi's report, which states that the knowledge of local history and geography was extremely poor among children of these NFE's. Hence, there is an urgent need to emphasize and rectify this aspect of education

H. Age-wise Rehabilitation

Since, the children of different age groups have different abilities of comprehension and cognition, it is necessary to provide them age-wise education. The classroom with children of varying age groups becomes chaotic and hampers learning. This is also true in relation to other activities like vocational training. So, the age factor should be considered while devising the plan for the rehabilitation of children.

I. Identity of its Own

Although, NFE schools were initiated to fulfill the absence of formal schools still they should not be taken as poor substitute of formal schools. These NFE have their own objective and characteristics and thus, have their own identity. This underlying uniqueness of its nature does not hinder the linkage with the formal schools and institutions, but in fact provides alternative entry points to these institutions or systems.

J. The Criteria of Replicability

Only such models of NFE should be developed which can be replicated. Hence, one should not encourage efforts which are basically resource intensive and do not have underlying structure which can be replicated elsewhere.

K. Skill Development

There should be clarity on the emphasis of education that should be skill building. The education can be on reading, writing and vocational, business or commercial skills. This becomes more important in the existing condition because the poor children do not have long time period for education like upper and middle class children.

L. Human Rights Education

Children should be made aware of their rights as children and as human beings. They should be encouraged to participate in the demonstrations organised by the implementing NGOs. This way they could learn to assert their rights and can understand the power of collective bargaining.

M. Establishment of Libraries

Along with the NFE, a parallel process of establishing a small library commensurate with learning level of children, should be made for promoting self-learning (sustainability) chances in these children. Some of the students may join formal schools after NFEs or some would like to end their education after that, but still there would be children who would like to continue their learning process on their own. These libraries can be established with the help of governmental schemes available for this purpose—these libraries can be managed by village education committee with the help of expertise available with local NGOs. The government can provide funds to NGO or a registered Village Education Committee after successful completion of NFE.

N. Teachers Selection

Teachers should be selected as far as possible from the same socio-cultural region. These teachers should be trained to appreciate the local language and concept, and utilise it in teaching children.

The language of instruction should be, as far as possible, the mother tongue of the children.

Conclusion

These are just suggestions which have emerged during restricted interaction with a small group of people and my experiences as the co-coordinator, of the programme. So, naturally, these suggestions represent the consensus of a small group of people, which need not to be true in its entirety. But the underlying idea is to appeal to all parties for improving and strengthening NFE's. All of us i.e. government, NGOs, National and international organisations and individuals, should try to contribute in whatever way is possible for the betterment of rehabilitation process and in creating a situation where all children can get opportunity for their development and thus not compelled to join the labour force at an early age. A collaborative effort from all the concerned parties will provide maximum benefits to the deprived children. The time has come when these children should not be considered as an exclusive property of their family. The poverty of the family should not interfere in the growth of the child as there are adequate resources in the world, of which even a small percentage is far enough, to get the basic amenities for development of proper health and education system. For instance, the *Human Development Report 1998* states that "... additional cost of achieving and maintaining universal access to basic education for all, basic health care for all, reproductive health care for all women, adequate food for all and safe water and sanitation for all is roughly $ 40 billion a year. This is less than 4% of the combined wealth of the 225 richest people in the world."

Reference

1. Zutshi, B. (1998): *An Assessment of Non Formal Education for the Freed Children from Carpet Weaving in Mirzapur-Bhadhoi , Project sponsored by REHA and SACCS.*

14

Alternative Learning a Child-Responsive and Community: Bhadhoi-Mirzapur Experiences

The UNICEF Approach : Bal Adhikar Pariyojana

1. Introduction

The Bal Adhikar Pariyojana is an integrated community-based initiative on the prevention of child labour. The Department of Women & Child Development, Govt. of U.P., is implementing it, with support from UNICEF. The project was launched on 15 August 1997 and is proposed to cover the core districts/blocks of the Bhadohi-Mirzapur carpet belt over a 5-year period.

As of June 1999, a total of 342 Gram Sabhas in four blocks in these two districts (total population: 800,000 approx.) are being covered.

While the long-term objective of the project is the elimination of child labour, the focus is on strategies to prevent children from joining the workforce. To achieve this, environment-building on Child Rights at various levels (village/panchayat/ block/district) is an integral intervention; this is supported by strengthened community partnership and organization towards demand generation and better utilization of existing services at the grassroots level.

Experice of Nalanda (Uttar Pradesh)

Nalanda is a U.P.-based resource centre for primary education. Its main aim is to provide technical support to both government and non-government agencies, working in the area of primary education. As part of its activities, the Centre is also involved in providing technical support for curriculum and materials development, research, planning, implementation of project plans, etc.

Nalanda is committed to quality improvement in primary education and at present, is associated with the alternative learning components of two major initiatives in the State--the Bal Adhikar Pariyojana, supported by UNICEF and the District Primary Education Project (DPEP), supported by the World Bank. Nalanda has been associated with the alternative learning component of the Bal Adhikar Pariyojana for over 18 months and is providing technical support in the areas of identification/selection and training of instructors, development of curriculum and materials, as well as monitoring & evaluation.

2. Promoting the Child's Right to Development

In accordance with its objectives, the Bal Adhikar Pariyojana focuses on making the Right to Development a goal of the community--the foundation for the holistic development of children lies in the quality of education and recreation that they receive. It is accepted that overcrowded government schools, shortage of teachers and lack of resources have had a serious impact on the quality of education, which has been further exacerbated by the uninteresting teaching-learning environment. As a result of this situation, combined with other social factors, children and education are getting further apart. Keeping this in mind, initiatives to promote children's right to quality education have been taken up by the Project.

3. The Situation

With a view to understand the primary education scenario in the project area, in terms of access to and the quality of schooling, as well as community/social perceptions on the value of education and develop integrated strategies to address the problem, the Bal Adhikar Pariyojana has facilitated assessments at various levels:

(a) PLA Community-based assessment has shown that—

- Although, in the project area, each Nyaya Panchayat has one or more primary schools, these are generally not accessible to those deprived/backward communities, who need them the most. Moreover, in many cases, schools are located far away from villages/hamlets which have a high proportion of SC/ST population.
- As per block-level data, 77 per cent boys and 61 per cent girls in the age group 6-11 years have been enrolled in school. Of those not attending school, a high proportion belongs to socio-economically backward communities and hardly any efforts have been made for their enrolment in formal school. It has also been noted that of the total enrolled children, 56 percent are attending private schools, and most of them belong to socially and economically better-off families.
- The following are the prime motivating factors contributing to the enrolment of children of the weaker communities
  - First mid-day meal
  - Second scholarship
  - Third Negligible fees
- Low enrolment, dependence of poor families on the child's income and the demand for child labour are the principal factors contributing the high dropout rates in school.
- An analysis of family expenditure pattern for education is given below:
  - Families with marginal income level 6% of total income
  - Families of middle-income level 8% of total income
  - Families of high income level 20% of total income

(b) Bat Garna (Child Database)

After the initial 6-month environment-building exercise, a village-level 'bal garna' was undertaken through local motivators covering all households and focussing on children 03-14 years.

An analysis of the data indicates that approximately 20 per cent of all the children in the age group of 6-14 years, are not in school. Of these, about 70 per cent are girls. Of that not in school, 90 per cent belong to SC/ST and backward communities. Of that not in school, an estimated 89 per cent have never been enrolled, while 11 per cent are dropouts. From the community perspective, the main reasons for non-enrolment are: (i) poverty and (ii) distance of school; involvement of girls in household chores has also been given as one of the main reasons for non-enrolment/dropouts.

However, a closer scrutiny at the family level has shown that, it is not the financial status of a family, but other societal norms and the perceived value of education that influence whether or not children are in school.

- Some families belonging to deprived communities are sending their children to school, while children belonging to higher caste families living in the same village/hamlet are not enrolled;
- Lower income/daily wage families are educating their children, while those with higher income levels are not sending their children to school
- For a particular family, poverty and the distance of the school are not impediments to educating their son, while the same factors are given as reasons for not educating their daughter

(c) Partnership with Women's Self-Help Groups (SHGs)

Regular discussions on the above issues relating to education take place with the SHGs, which have been organised in all villages covered under the Project. From such interaction, it has become evident that most families do not consider education necessary for their daily lives and the holistic development of their children. Irregular teaching in schools, and the perception that after being educated, the person will have higher aspirations and may not be inclined to work as a labourer further corroborates this attitude.

To address the above issues, the following action points have been taken up by the Project:

- Environment-building at the community-level on the critical importance of education
- Strengthening the process of enrolment/retention in schools
- Addressing the primary education needs of out-of-reach children
- Addressing factors which prohibit/prevent children from

entering mainstream formal school
- Reducing the dependence of families on children's income, viz. reduction in child labour

4. The Strategy

The following strategies are being implemented by the Bal Adhikar Pariyojana to address the education needs of children and influence community perceptions on the value of education:

(a) Community-level Environment-building—Project 'Utsah'

Through teams of local motivators, using folk media and interpersonal communication, village-level sensitisation on Child Rights is undertaken to bring about attitudinal change among communities and encourage their partnership in the project. During this 4-6 month intensive exercise, the linkages between child labour and illiteracy (lack of education) are explored, and popular myths relating to child labour discussed

- Illiteracy perpetuates poverty; it is not poverty, which contributes to lack of education
- Instead of contributing to family income, a working child deprives an adult in the family of much higher (adult) wages, as a result of which the total income of the family is decreased.

(b) Bal Garna

The Bal Garna is not merely an enumeration exercise; it is a process of identification of all school-going and non-school going children in the age group 3-14 years, ratio of boys: girls in each category, reasons for dropout, community perceptions on education, supplemented with information on the education and economic level of their parents. By including children in 3-6 age group, an attempt has been made to identify children for early childhood education and school readiness initiatives.

(c) Convergence with the Education Department

The Project has established linkages with the Government's basic Shiksha Department. The outcomes of the community mobilization activities and the 'Bal Garna' have been discussed with the Department in detail, to promote synergy and convergence and avoid duplication of effort. The following joint efforts have been initiated

'School Chalo' Abhivaan (school enrolment drive)

A school enrolment drive is launched annually in July in all the villages covered by the Project. The strategy is finalised after detailed discussions with participants at the block-level meeting of Principals of primary schools held at the Block Resource Centre, as also with the NGO partners.

The highlights of the strategy are as follows:

- Information dissemination and social mobilization through wall writings, posters and pamphlets.
- Village-level meetings (one meeting covering two villages) with involvement of the community, gram panchayat representatives, Members of the Village Education Committee, representative of the Education Department, and other local leaders, to ensure their participation in the campaign.
- Motivation of all families identified with non-school going children (basis: Bal Garna) to enrol their children in the formal school catering to that village.
- Facilitate interaction between parents and school to promote enrolment of all children.

Follow-up of Enrolled Children

After the conclusion of the 'School Chalo Abhiyaan' (31 July) regular follow-up of the enrolled children, especially potential dropouts, is undertaken by the Project for the entire academic session (i.e. up to March the following year). This involves:

- Identification of children with irregular/non-attendance (with the help of local motivators).
- At village-level weekly meetings, interaction with families of such children on reasons for irregular/non attendance.
- Attempt to resolve bottlenecks which act as impediments to attendance (family and school level).
- At the end of the academic session, the school certifies the

number of children with regular attendance. This provides up-to-date feedback on the follow-up actions taken by the project.

5. Alternative Learning

Despite the above efforts to mainstream children into formal primary school, there are still children who are out-of-reach of the formal school system due to socio-economic reasons. To address the educational needs of such children, 69 Alternative Learning Centres (ALCs), covering 2,651 children between 6-12 years, have been operational to-date under the Project. The strategy adopted is as follows:

- Identification of all non-school going children especially working children and girls ('bal garna').
- Identification of potential instructors (one ALC of 40 children) in collaboration with the local panchayat and community.
- Selection and training of the instructors in collaboration with the Basic Education Department and Nalanda Resource Centre.
- Space arrangements for the ALCs to be provided by the local Panchayat and community.
- Ongoing monitoring of the ALCs (attendance of children and instructor, teaching/learning activities, etc) to be done by the SHGs and local Panchayat.
- Classroom transaction: four *hours/day* (timings to be determined by the community); learning achievement up to Class V to be completed in three years (six semesters (Entry Phase-cum-Introduction + Class IV) of six months each); mainstreaming of children into formal school as and when appropriate i.e. when specific minimum levels of learning achieved
- Child-centred, rapid, multigrade, activity-based teaching/ learning curriculum and materials (Textbooks-cum-workbooks), focussing on achievement of minimum levels of learning, developed by Nalanda to be use by the ALCs.
- The ALCs status as on April 1999 was:
  - 69 ALCs in operation covering two phase I blocks.
  - Total children registered: 2651

- 35-40 children per ALC
- 96% of children enrolled are first generation learners.

6. Selection of Instructors

This is the first step in the ALC operationalisation process. The Gram Pradhan is requested to provide three names of potential candidates, based on the following criteria:

- Minimum educational level: Class X
- Of the three candidates, mandatory for one each from SC/ST and backward communities
- Priority given to women candidates
- Candidates are expected to be child-friendly and create a conducive environment for learning

On receiving the nominations, a 1-day workshop is organised to which all the applicants are invited and through various objective techniques, their skills and capacities (specific focus on language and maths) are assessed and especially their ability to interact with children.

Based on this assessment, the applicant who scores the highest among the three per village is short-listed. These short listed candidates are then given an intensive 10-day Foundation Training during which their performance is once again assessed. If found suitable they are then given the responsibility for running an ALC.

Nalanda has developed a module on the detailed process to be followed for instructor selection.

7. Curriculum Design

Development of curriculum for Alternative Learning is the mainstay of Nalanda's collaboration with the Bal Adhikar Pariyojana. The challenge was to develop a curriculum, which would address the diverse learning needs of different age groups of children attending the ALC, with focus on pedagogy and teaching/learning skills.

To facilitate this, Nalanda carried out a situation-cum-needs assessment in the project area. Interaction with parents indicated that the lack of quality primary education in government schools was one of the main reasons why children are not enrolled. In addition, if parents can readily see the positive impact of quality education on their children, they will ensure regular attendance.

Keeping these factors in mind, the curriculum to be developed needed to be:

(i) Interesting for the child,
(ii) Contextually relevant and applicable to the local environment, and
(iii) Facilitating rapid learning.

Moreover, key aspects such as 'learning-by-doing' i.e. experiential learning, stimulation, etc. have been integrated into the curriculum. Thus, the curriculum is 'process-centred' and not based on note learning and incorporates local-specific stories, poems, etc.

It was also felt that the curriculum should be such that it is not alien to the children's environment but gets easily integrated into their daily lives. In most instances, the relevance of the curriculum to the children's environment is not considered important. As a result, the curriculum usually becomes uninteresting and meaningless and does not stimulate children's enthusiasm. Thus, in order to awaken children's curiosity, it is important to include elements that stimulate the thinking process. The ALC curriculum developed under the Project attempts to address these critical aspects.

The teaching/learning materials developed by Nalanda are in conformity with the norms set by the Government for Class I to Class V and are based on the minimum levels of learning stipulated by NCERT. In addition, children are given several opportunities for experimentation and developing their imagination. For example, the pictures in the workbooks are only outlines; the children can fill in the colours themselves.

In short, it can be said that the materials developed are not only informative and educative, but are also child-oriented and provide ample opportunity for children to develop their aptitudes and skills.

(a) Entry-level Curriculum

The curriculum being developed for the ALCs covers a period of three years. An 'entry-level' curriculum has been designed for the first 3-months with the objective of creating a facilitating and attractive learning environment for children and make them the habit to come to school. This is important, since 96 per cent of the children attending the ALCs are first-generation learners.

The curriculum is based on the elements of 'joyful learning' and includes an introduction to language, maths and environment and has been found to be very useful in promoting a child-friendly approach to learning.

(b) Language

It was observed that, initially, all children attending the ALCs speak the local dialect and are not familiar with standard Hindi. This is not considered an impediment to the teaching/learning process and children are given full freedom to express themselves as they wish. This has helped develop a close link between the children and the centre and contributed to regular attendance.

It was also felt that language textbooks usually do not give importance to the child's thinking and expression abilities—they are more factual and didactic, with no relevance to the child's world. Moreover, the teachers also expect that the textbooks include question-answers, which the children can learn by note and reproduce during the examinations. As a result, the fundamental thinking process of the child is not given due recognition while designing textbooks. The workbooks developed by Nalanda attempt to address this critical issue.

(c) Maths

The idea of 'concepts' is crucial to a well-designed maths curriculum. Therefore, at the initial stage, children need to be given solid objects to handle so that they understand shapes through learning-by-doing. Subsequently, visuals and concepts need to be introduced. It has generally be observed that in most maths textbooks, children are introduced to various concepts too early and too quickly which, in fact, they are not mentally ready for and therefore, cannot understand or grasp. These considerations have been kept in mind while designing the workbooks under the Project. In addition, more importance is given to the process rather than the end result.

(d) Environmental Studies

The EVS curriculum is designed in such a manner so as to provide an opportunity to children to better understand their environment. Thus, it includes such components with which children can easily identify, self-experiment and eventually draw inferences from. Thus, EVS should not merely provide information/knowledge, but also develop the proficiency and skills of the child.

(e) Multigrade Teaching

Since the ALCs cater to a range of age groups 6-14 years, there was a need to develop material, which would address the educational needs of this wide range of children and, at the same time, hold the interest of each and every child.

As a result, textbooks-cum-workbooks have been designed which are easy-to-use and encourage creativity. Moreover, for Classes I & II, these textbooks-cum-workbooks (language and maths) have been divided into three units and two units, respectively, to take care of the pace of learning of different age groups.

8. Instructor's Training

Development of child- responsive curriculum is not enough-- in fact, it is much more important to ensure that the teaching/learning process at the ALCs is effective, for which instructor training is crucial. More often than not, it is observed that since the instructors themselves have been taught using the relational method, it is difficult for them to accept the child responsive methods and translate these into teaching skills. Here again, learning-by-doing forms the basis of instructor training, which is also participatory to ensure full involvement of the trainees.

Instructors' training is perceived as an educational process—its objective is not only to promote creativity, knowledge and information as well as skills development but, more importantly, stimulate the thinking process of the participants. It is, therefore, a continuous process, which guides and inspires both the trainer and trainee to share experiences and widen their horizons.

Generally, in most training it is expected that the trainer is the repository of knowledge and that he knows it all. In such a situation, the trainee is merely a passive recipient. To make such trainings more meaningful, the active participation of the trainee is ensured through sharing of experiences and learning from each other.

(a) Foundation Training

The Foundation Training covers a period of 10 days and includes the following topics:

- Concept of alternative learning
- Principles of child- responsive teaching/learning
- Curriculum
- Pedagogy
- Management of ALCs participatory techniques to ensure community participation

The entire training is process-oriented using different simulation and motivation techniques.

(b) Refresher Training

Refresher trainings are held at 6-monthly intervals and focus on specific topics based on the textbooks/workbooks. This is supplemented by problem-solving sessions during which practical solutions to field-level problems, faced by the instructors, in running the ALCs, are discussed.

In addition, a monthly meeting of ALC instructors is also convened to review the lesson plan for the previous month, discuss the lesson plan for the following month and resolve problems.

9. Assessment

Periodic assessment is an essential tool to determine the progress of children attending the ALCs. Such assessments are activity-based and carried out in a child-friendly atmosphere so that the children do not feel that they are under any pressure to perform. Parents should be also requested to ensure that their children are present at the ALC during this time. Through the assessment, it is ensured that each child achieves an acceptable level of proficiency (as defined in the curriculum), before moving on to the next level and being given the upgraded set of textbooks/ workbooks.

The *Entry-level/Introductory curriculum* is for a period of three months during which a monthly assessment of levels of learning/ skills is carried out for each child.

The subsequent levels (Class I to Class V) are for duration of six months each, for which the textbooks/workbooks are divided into two/three units. Assessments are carried out every time a child completes one unit and is ready to move on to the next. Such a process is, therefore, sensitive to the different pace of learning of each child and acts, as a guide to the instructor on the specific learning needs of each child. It is emphasised that the focus should be more on the process of assessment, rather than the end result and that such a. process is in-built into the functioning of the ALC.

10. Management of ALCs

It is most challenging to implement an education initiative--to meet this challenge it is essential that the Project Management Unit has an in-depth understanding, not only of what is meant by quality education, but also of the principles and processes of child-responsive teaching/learning.

To facilitate this process, a 5-day orientation of the PMU was organised during which the entire gamut of topics relating to education, both formal and alternative, were discussed. Based on the outcomes, an Operations Manual has been developed which serves as a guide to the entire process of ALC operationalisation-selection of villages, identification/selection of instructors, training methodology/techniques, monitoring, supervision, evaluation as well as community participation.

11. Monitoring

Monitoring plays a critical role for the success of any project. Keeping this in mind, an effective monitoring system has been developed, detailing the specific responsibilities at various levels—from village up to the district. Using this system, information on each ALC is available through different sources and can be cross-checked, thereby leaving no scope for incorrect information.

At the village-level, the women SHGs (which are an integral component of the Project) review the functioning of the ALC at their weekly meeting. Since children from the families of these women are attending the ALCs, they have a personal interest in the regular functioning of the centre and are, therefore, in a position to provide reality-based feedback to the local motivators.

The motivators, themselves, also spend some time at the ALC during their weekly visit to the village and maintain regular contact with the parents. As a result, feedback on the ALCs is discussed at the weekly meeting of the motivators at which the PMU is also present.

12. Supervision

One local supervisor has been identified for 15 centres and is expected to visit every ALC under her/his charge at least twice a month. The supervision responsibilities include:

- Review attendance and day-to-day functioning;
- Assess learning levels of children;
- Discuss/resolve problems;
- Contact parents of those children with **low/non attendance** and motivate them to re-send their wards;
- Take corrective action, as appropriate.

The supervisor is also responsible to set up a Parents' Committee at the village level and convene monthly meetings at which progress and problems of the ALCs can be discussed. The outcomes of such meetings are included in the monthly report submitted by the Supervisor to the Project Management Unit (PMU) of the Bal Adhikar Pariyojana.

The PMU team is also responsible for ALC monitoring on a monthly basis, with greater attention being paid to those centres facing problems and taking corrective action as and when required.

In addition to the above, one resource person from Nalanda devotes six days/month for technical monitoring in the project area. The first day is devoted to meeting the PMU and the supervisors at which the monthly progress is reviewed, technical problems addressed and follow-up discussions held, followed by a visit to problematic centres. Random visits to other centres is also undertaken during which the indicators listed above are assessed. The monitoring reports are submitted to the PMU and appropriate corrective action taken accordingly.

Such intensive monitoring is considered essential, at least in the initial phase of ALC operationalisation, since it helps streamline the process and address critical issues relating to teaching/learning, which in the long run, would be beneficial to the project.

13. Alternative Learning Centres: Special

Features

- Goal: Enrolment of all children 6+ into formal primary school in the project area within a period of five years

- Duration: 4 hours between 0 a.m. 10 a.m. to 4 p.m.
- 35-40 children/centre.
- Mobilization of communities to promote education as the main tool for poverty eradication.
- Inculcate, within communities, the value and importance of quality education as opposed to mid-day meal and scholarship.
- Promote community level monitoring through panchayats, women SHGs and parents' committees.
- Active convergence with the Basic Education Department.
- Mainstreaming of those children who have attained levels of learning in the ALCs into formal primary school; inclusion of new children from the village into the ALCs.
- Multigrade teaching based on child- responsive curriculum.

The Carpet Belt of Bhadhoi-Mirzapur, Uttar Pradesh

Objective

The overall objective of the project is the prevention of child labour. Advocating, implementing and monitoring programme approaches which are multi-sectoral and converge on families and communities which are 'at risk' of putting their children to work.

Thus, the two underlying issues being addressed by the Bal Adhikar Pariyojana are:

- Denial of children's rights, especially the right to education and protection from exploitation and abuse;
- Cycle of poverty-debt-illiteracy-unemployment.

With greater emphasis and focus on the prevention of child labour, the project also envisages selected inputs to complement and supplement ongoing government and other efforts relating to rehabilitation.

Coverage

Project initiated in August 1997.

Over a 5-year period, intensive coverage of two core districts of Bhadohi and Mirzapur, covering a total population of approx. 2,700,000, of which about 25 per cent are marginalized, i.e. belong to scheduled castes or other backward classes. In addition, the carpet-intensive blocks from adjacent districts of Varanasi, Jaunpur and Allahabad will also be covered.

Phasing

- From October 1997 to May 1998, the following four development blocks have been taken up under the project, covering a population of approx. 800,000 spread over 303 village clusters:

Period	*Bhadohi*	*Mirzapur*	*Gram Sabhas*	*Population*
Oct.'97-Aug. 98	Aurai block	Chhanbe	109	250,000
		Block.	92	200,000
Sep.'98-Aug.'99	Bhadohi	Majhwa	103	220,000
			38	130,000

- Due to the time-intensive nature of the project, there is usually a 'gestation period' of 6 to 8 months during which community needs assessment and prioritisation (through participatory techniques), followed by intensive environment building-cum-social mobilization at the community/village level is undertaken. 'Visible' project activities are initiated only after rapport-building and community participation is ensured. This period is, therefore, critical to lay the foundation on which project activities in a particular village can be built.
- Thus, expansion of coverage to new blocks takes place every 8 to 9 months.

Activities

Participatory Learning and Action (PLA).

The broad results of PLA conducted in the two Phase I blocks (Aurai and Chhanbe) indicate that debt-poverty--illiteracy cycle is the major cause for children being involved in labour; in fact, approx. 30 per cent of the total family income comes from credit (at usurious rates of interest) to meet consumption needs.

The PLA exercises conducted in the two Phase II block (Bhadohi and Majhwa), from December 1998 to January 1999, show similar findings.

Environment-building Project 'Utsah'

- In partnership with NG0s, environment-building is an integral component of the Bal Adhikar Pariyojana; to date, four NG0s—Sarifa, Gramras, Sneha and Saarthak—are collaborating with the project in the Phase I and II blocks.
- The NGOs are responsible for co-ordinating as well as monitoring the field-level work of a total of 120 local motivators (a team of two motivators for every five villages).
- After the initial 4-month intensive rapport-building exercise in each block, the motivators continue to act as the link between the community and the project (see box).

Motivators: Roles and Responsibilities

- Rapport-building with communities and information dissemination on the objectives/goals of the project.
- Maintain regular contact (once-a-month) with Gram Pradhan, Panchayat members, primary school teacher, health worker (ANM), Anganwadi worker and other village leaders.
- Convene one community meeting every month to discuss common problems and issues.
- Inform community on fixed day for immunization (day/ date, location, time and name of ANM); ensure complete immunization for all children 0-2 years.
- Identify pregnant women and promote TT immunization, antenatal checkups and referral (in collaboration with ANM).
- Inform community about diarrhoea management (use of ORS and HAF); act as ORS depot holders.
- Identify all children in the age group of 6-14 that are out of school and facilitate their enrolment and retention.
- Monitor functioning of alternate learning centres (attendance of children and instructor, community participation, availability and use of teaching/learning material).
- Mobilise women for the formation and activation of SHGs,

including monitoring of savings, bank linkages and inter-group loaning.
- Initiate and promote dialogue within SHGs on key social issues affecting women and children, especially the girl child.
- Provide reliable feedback to the Project Management Unit (through the NGOs) for appropriate action.

Primary Education

'School Chalo Abhiyaan' (campaign for primary school enrolment) followed by *'Retention Drives'*
- Initiated in June-July 1998 in 100 villages of Phase I blocks, through 67 village-level meetings with participation of 7,366 persons—panchayat representatives, village education committee (VEC), members, education department officials, local opinion leaders and communities
- 3,100 children (6-12 years—1,568 boys and 1,332 girls) enrolled in government primary schools. Active follow-up on their retention being done in collaboration with VECs as well as local motivators
- As of 31 March 1999, of the 3,100 children enrolled, 2,625 (87%) are regularly attending school
- The campaign will be an on-going activity to be carried out in all blocks in the months of June-July every year, so that eligible children get into the mainstream education process.

Bal Garna (child database)

- The *'school chalo abhiyaan'* is supplemented by a *'bal garna'*-- a village level database to ascertain the status of primary education in the project area; this data collection exercise covers household information on

  (a) Family size, disaggregated by age and gender;
  (b) Income and main occupation of family, including that of children;
  (c) Education level/school participation status.

- In 1998, the *'bal garna'* was completed in 109 villages of Phase I blocks; it has been initiated in 150 villages of Phase II blocks in April 1999 *and was expected to be completed by June 1999.*

Alternate Learning Centres (ALCs)

Based on the *'bal garna'*, alternative learning centres (ALCs) have been operational. Based on the spatial mapping exercise undertaken, it is estimated that 75 ALCs will be established every year

Criteria

1. Village not covered by primary school.
2. Large number of out-of-school children, including the working child.

Salient Features

- Local instructor selected by the community and trained by a resource team (Nalanda).
- Child responsive curriculum and methods used.
- Textbooks and workbooks developed by Nalanda based on existing government curriculum, but adapted to fit into the cultural milieu of the child.
- Ongoing assessment of each child so that once a certain level of school readiness is reached, the child is mainstreamed into the formal school system.
- Regular contact with the VECs and the Government's Basic Education Department to facilitate mainstreaming.

ALC Status (April 1999)

- 69 ALCs in operation covering two Phase 1 blocks
- Total children registered: 2,651
- 35-40 children per ALC
- 96% of children enrolled are first generation learners

Women's Empowerment

Participation of women in the development process, especially in the area of thrift/credit linked to economic viability, is a critical strategy to address the debt-poverty cycle, which is one of the principal root causes of child labour. The process of mobilising women from the project villages to form self-help groups (SHGs) was initiated in January 1998 (Aurai block) and in September 1998 (Chhanbe block), facilitated by a technical resource group, Saarthi Development Foundation. Intensive field-based training, in five phases, was carried out during which the SHGs were linked to nationalised banks and inter-group loaning process initiated.

As of April 1999,

- 184 SHGs were operationalised.
- The SHGs had a membership of 2,058 women (*Note:* one prerequisite for membership is that all children from the woman's family should be in school).
- Monthly savings ranging from Rs. 10/- to Rs. 40/- per member (depending on the SHG).
- Total savings per month for all the SHGs is approx. Rs. 22,670/- in Aurai and Rs. 10,735 in Chhanbe blocks.
- 109 bank accounts opened in Aurai block, with a total savings of Rs. 181,000.
- Inter-group loaning commenced in January 1999 in 55 groups in Aurai block,' with a total of Rs. 72,840 being revolved as loans.
- A total of 191 women have taken loans for the following purposes.

  1. To pay off earlier debt to the local moneylender (rate of interest charged by the groups ranges from 2 to 3 per cent per month, as against the moneylenders' interest rate of 10 to 12 per cent per month).
  2. Towards school books/other costs.
  3. Towards medicine.
  4. Towards wedding/festival expenses.
  5. Towards small micro enterprises (vegetable vending, etc).

Viable Economic Opportunities

In collaboration with STEP foundation (Swiss Consortium of Carpet Importers), a women's Training-Cum-Production Centre (TCPC) for carpet weaving has been established in Gharnhapur village in Aurai block and 24 women from two SHGs mobilized under the project are being provided training in high-quality carpet weaving through a local exporter, M/s. Triveni Carpets. The infrastructure costs are being met through STEP Foundation, while the training component is being funded through the Bal Adhikar Pariyojana. On completion of the training, the local exporter has agreed to directly liaison with the women for production of carpets and marketing/export to Switzerland. It is hoped that this pilot initiative, launched on 01 April 1999, will pave the way for similar collaborative efforts in other villages in the area and, more importantly, demonstrate the viability of 'women's co-operatives' in this critical sector of the village economy.

Similar viable income-generation opportunities are being explored for other SHGs with institutional finance (NABARD and the District Rural Industries Project, Mirzapur), and linkages to government anti-poverty and employment-generation schemes such as MCRA, Indira Mahila Yojana (IMY), Rashtriya Mahila Kosh (RMK), etc.

Availability-cum-market survey has also been undertaken by the technical resource agency, and several micro-enterprises identified for SHG linkages; SDS training for capacity-building of the women will be supported under the project while start-up/ revolving funds will be generated through the tasks.

Sustainability of SHGs as Community-based Organizations (CBOs)

The SHGs have gradually started monitoring project implementation at the village level for the children, who have been enrolled in formal schools. The purpose:

- To see the ALC instructor are regular.
- Is *teaching/learning* taking place? Are all the children who have been enrolled regular at the ALC?
- If not, one of the SHG members, personally contacts the family to find out the reasons for non-attendance.
- Is the health worker (ANM) visiting the health centre as per schedule?
- Is immunization being given free of cost? Are the families with eligible infants availing the service?

Appropriate capacity-building strategies are being adopted to ensure gradual transfer of responsibilities for project implementation to the SHGs.

Partnerships and Networking

Panchayats

In view of the increasing devolution of powers to local governments Panchayats, the project continues to dialogue with Panchayat representatives, especially the Gram Pradhan and the BDC members.

So far, 75 formal meetings, covering all four blocks, have been organised for the elected representatives on the objectives of the project, seeking their involvement and support in project implementation and monitoring. The outcomes have been mixed. While support has been forthcoming in these villages in terms of provision of Panchayat land for the ALC, or the construction of the training-cum-production centre, or even liaisoning with the block functionaries for basic services, in some areas, especially those where the caste/class differences are more striking. These issues are being addressed constructively as part of the overall project strategy.

Carpet Manufacturers

Regular interaction is also taking place with the carpet manufacturers' associations, the Carpet Export Promotion Council (CEPC) and the All India Carpet Manufacturers' Association (AICMA) on issues of mutual interest.

Rugmark Foundation

The Rugmark Foundation has also sought the project's collaboration in training a batch of 25 instructors from their schools in child responsive teaching/learning methodology

The PMU team visited child labour initiatives, both government and NGO, in the States of Andhra Pradesh and Tamil Nadu in February 1999. This visit was an excellent learning opportunity for the team and facilitated the exchange of ideas and experiences between U.P. and the other States.

Going Beyond

The local-level networks (NG0s and motivators) have been actively collaborating with on-going national/state government campaigns in the areas of health, viz.

- Pulse Polio 1998—a total of 30,511 children (0-5 years) were immunised at booths manned by the project teams
- NNT
- Diarrhoea Management (the SHGs and motivators have been given the responsibility by the Health Department as ORS depot holders)

The ALCs and SHGs have also been mobilized to participate in special events such as Republic Day (26 January) and Women's Day (8 March)

Project Monitoring

- An integrated Management Information System (MIS)—community up to State-level—is in the process of being developed and field-tested. It is expected that this MIS will focus on both qualitative and quantitative aspects and facilitate two-way feedback for effective project implementation and monitoring.
- The Project Management Unit (PMU) is at the core of project planning, implementation and monitoring and liases with the district administrations, NG0s, UNICEF and other partners.
- The PMU reports on project progress to the Divisional-level Steering Committee chaired by the Divisional Commissioner, which meets bi-monthly.
- The State-level Steering Committee, chaired by the Secretary, Dept. of Women and Child Development, Govt. of UP, meets every quarter.

15

RUGMARK: Campaign against Child Labour

S. Sondhi

Most of us present in this seminar have happy memories of a joyful childhood, spent in the warmth of our parent's love and affection; playing happily with our childhood companions; studying at reputed, well equipped schools in the company of our friends. It is so tempting to want to believe that all children are able to lead similar, happy childhood. But, unfortunately for millions of poor children forced to work, a happy childhood is only a distant dream. Worse still, the real life for these children turns into a nightmare of long unending hours of hard labour subsisting on the barest minimum of nourishment and every now and then reaping the reward of brutal corporal punishment at the hands of their employers.

It is incredible that more than a century after abolishing slavery, our modern world has been unable to set our children free from the clutches of bondage and forced labour. All our economic prosperity, growth and progress of science and technology remains of scarce importance and use, if children remain uneducated and are exploited. All the progress of science and technology will be of no use for minds which are uneducated and scarred by traumas of forced labour suffered during childhood.

The factors universally and unanimously identified as the root cause for child labour have been poverty and illiteracy. But an equally potent cause for the perpetuation of child labour is the absence of an alternative opportunity for their rehabilitation. Different governments all over the world have promulgated strict laws against use of child labour. But the problem continues to worsen. The problem continues to deteriorate because the 'anti-child-labour laws', in the absence of strict enforcement, lack the teeth to evoke compliance from its worst offenders and also fail to provide an alternative to children from working. Most of these laws remain ineffective and unpopular in the absence of an holistic approach towards the liberation and rehabilitation of child labour.

India is stated to have the largest number of urban and rural child workers in the world. The official figure for working children, based on the National Sample Survey conducted in 1987-88, is placed at 17.5 million. While the estimates by various organisation range from 44 million to over 100 million child workers.

Child labour is not an isolated problem, there is not a single remedy or "magic bullet". It cannot be eradicated overnight by a single government order. Nor will it disappear, because one or more company decides to sack its child workers, or even if all the countries of the industrialised world agree not to buy goods made by children. Putting an end to child labour requires a package of changes and is bound to take some time. It requires a general improvement in the economy of the country, a reduction in the gap between the rich and poor, improvement in a country's educational infrastructure and efforts to promote awareness of the need for change.

Major export industries in India which are said to utilise child labour include hand-knotted carpets, gemstone polishing, brass and base metal articles, glass and glassware, footwear, textiles and silk, and fireworks. However the exact number of child workers engaged in these industries is not known. It is only on the basis of estimates that people have tried to quantify the presence of child labour in these industries. Nevertheless the presence, and exploitation, of child labour in the carpet industry is well noted. This is despite the existence of "Employment of Children Act-1938", banning children from working in the carpet industry. This act has been followed by the "Child Labour (Prohibition and Regulation) Act passed in 1986. Though, the requisite laws to control such abuses have existed, but an adequate implementation has been lacking all along. Which is the reason that despite the law, abuses have persisted for decades and even grown worse in recent years under increased export pressure.

Hand-knotted carpet industry is one of the major exporting

and foreign exchange earning industry of India. These carpets are exported in large quantities to the United States and Germany. The value of exports achieved by this industry has been constantly on the rise, providing employment directly and indirectly to an ever-increasing number of people. Despite the importance of this industry, it has remained neglected and subject to apathy from concerned authorities to help to improve its image and save it from the stigma of child labour. Realising the urgency and necessity to take concrete steps in this direction RUGMARK was launched to limit the damage done to the industry by a much maligned image for engaging child labour and also to provide a marketing impetus to the Indian carpets in the world markets.

RUGMARK is one of the first initiative to provide a holistic approach to the removal and rehabilitation of child labour. Limited, presently, only to the carpet manufacturing industry, RUGMARK has evoked, over its four years of existence, an overall positive response. It is an Indian initiative, unique in its concept and transparent in its execution. It accords topmost priority to removal of child labour from carpet weaving and their suitable rehabilitation. Along side it ensures that the carpet trade, under threat of a possible ban by importing countries due to child labour issue and failing demand due to economic recession witnessed world-wide, does not suffer. Success of RUGMARK can also be judged from the fact that many other similar initiatives have been attempted, based on its principles and encouraged by its promising start.

The RUGMARK Foundation, a private, voluntary, non-profit entity incorporated in September 1994, consists of representatives of Development Organisations, manufacturers, exporters of carpets, and leading NGOs. This combination of various groups gives RUGMARK the necessary credibility in India and, in particular, the target markets. In no way does it seek to replace any government authority or act as a regulatory body in the carpet industry. RUGMARK has been effective largely due to the fact that it seeks to involve the constituents of the carpet industry in redressing its problems. In the present case, the constituents of the carpet industry importers, exporters, loom owners and weavers'--are all involved at different stages of the implementation of RUGMARK scheme.

The prime consideration behind the launch of RUGMARK was to offer an alternative to the consumers, who were likely to boycott carpets, made by child labour, under the influence of unrelenting and concerted crusade against child labour in the carpet industry, launched by various Indian NGOs, led by Mr. Kailash Satyarthi and supported by like-minded NG0s abroad. Hence, awareness about child labour was awakened at the same time as the framework for RUGMARK, as a visual guarantee for carpets without child labour, was being formulated. Support and contribution of the Indo German Export Promotion Project (IGEP), New Delhi in drawing up the blueprint for RUGMARK and its implementation has been exemplary.

RUGMARK is a marketing tool. It seeks help to maintain the carpet market and to increase export possibilities. RUGMARK provides an assurance to the consumers that the carpets carrying this label have been manufactured and exported by a company which has voluntarily committed itself to work without child labour and that the production facilities of this company during unannounced random inspection conducted by RUGMARK were seen and were not found employing individuals below 14 years of age.

Under RUGMARK the carpet exporter as well as production units commit themselves in legally binding manner not to employ children under 14 years in the production of carpets, and to pay their workers at least the official minimum wages. In the case of traditional family enterprises, children under 14 years assisting their parents in the job must attend school regularly.

The exporters make available to the RUGMARK Foundation, a complete list of looms and sources from which they procure their carpets. These lists are regularly updated. The exporters are bound to have their loom units and premises inspected by professional inspectors of the RUGMARK Foundation at any time without prior notice.

The compliance with the RUGMARK principles is monitored through inspections of the looms as well as the exporters' premises by professional inspectors who are employed and supervised by the RUGMARK Foundation. Additionally, NGOs working in the carpet producing areas monitor the commitment towards non-employment of child workers.

After the full compliance with the RUGMARK criteria, the right to use the RUGMARK label is granted to the respective exporter through a licence agreement, which defines the legal modalities for the use of the RUGMARK labels. Any deviation from the RUGMARK criteria will lead to the withdrawal of the right to use the RUGMARK label.

The RUGMARK is affixed on the carpets by those exporters who have obtained the right to use it. Each label carries an individual serial number through which each carpet can be traced back to its manufacturing/exporting unit by means of the RUGMARK database.

After establishing a credible inspection system to ensure the detection and removal of child labour from carpet weaving during the first year of its operations, RUGMARK accorded topmost priority to the other important aspect of its functioning, namely rehabilitation and education of child weavers. After undertaking detailed ground work to ensure a flawless launch and implementation of its educational and rehabilitation project, RUGMARK inaugurated in quick succession respectively in the months of August and October in 1996, a Primary School for weavers' children and a "Transitory Rehabilitation Centre" for children removed from carpet weaving. Both the projects are located in the carpet belt and functioning well. Our inspections and rehabilitation programmes are very closely inter-linked. Without one, the other is not possible.

BALASHRYA is the first major project by RUGMARK for the rehabilitation and education of child weavers removed from carpet weaving. BALASHRYA is a shelter, an abode for children who are freed from carpet weaving and need overall help to facilitate their reintegration into the mainstream of society. It is an integrated project, which provides these children lots of care and understanding besides education—both formal and non-formal, vocational training to learn a craft or trade, to become self-sufficient and develop a healthy attitude towards society and life. Presently housing 61 child weavers, out of whom 55 are bonded child labours.

Our keen desire to provide quality education to weavers' children and those removed from the looms, saw its realisation in the shape of RUGMARK Primary Schools, inaugurated in August 1996 and to day we have four primary schools catering to the needs of 950 children. The schools are located in the heart of the carpet belt and are functioning well to the entire satisfaction of all concerned. The children enrolled range from 6-13 years and most of who have never been to school earlier. Response of the villagers, exporters and above all the children enrolled, is extremely encouraging. Already people from other villages and many of our licensees are requesting us to open similar schools in other areas of the carpet belt. Incidentally, the buildings for two of our schools has been given by our licensees. The opening of the Primary Schools is not the end of the story. The parents of the children, motivated at the success of their wards, requested us to do something to educate them too. With the result, we are to day running six Adult Education Centres as adjuncts to our Primary Schools and providing education to 53 ladies and 137 men (all parents of children studying in our Schools and carpet weavers). The credit for the impetus and the need to open the Rehabilitation Centre and the schools goes to our Chairperson Mrs. Maneka Gandhi, who has been the guiding spirit behind these projects.

Although reaction of people to RUGMARK—its concept, aim and execution--has ranged from downright scepticism to indifference, but what even its most vociferous detractors cannot deny now is the definite and for-all-to-see contribution of RUGMARK in creating greater awareness in the carpet belt, among exporters, weavers and villagers, about the need to keep children away from carpet weaving and to provide them with education and alternative vocations. Contribution of RUGMARK is acknowledged without inhibition by foreign NGOs' representatives visiting India, importers and others related to the child labour issues.

Recently, closer home, even the Indian judiciary has passed the ruling, calling for a more active, practical and result-oriented approach towards addressing the problem of child labour. We are sure that as and when government machinery starts implementing the ruling of the judiciary, they would find in RUGMARK, an excellent and result-oriented example to emulate and base their efforts on. In the alternative they may also consider, in view of the unqualified success of RUGMARK during its short span of operations, to offer us full support and assistance to pursue and achieve our goal to make carpet weaving a child labour-free industry, a precursor to setting free other industries also of the stigma of child labour.

In conclusion, I would like to say that RUGMARK starting from very humble beginnings nearly four years ago, today has notched up most creditable statistics viz. 209 exporters licensed to use RUGMARK on their carpets made without child labour. During this period of hard, sincere and dedicated work, the RUGMARK inspection staff has been able to inspect about 52,157 looms and detected 782 looms with children. The total number of looms under RUGMARK are 25,347, while the number of children detected during inspection is 1257. Moreover the number of carpets for which RUGMARK labels has been issued is nearing 1.5 million mark. These figures reflect the success and efficacy of RUGMARK system and immense potential to help solve the problem of child labour.

16

Child Labour Rehabilitation Programmes—Experience of PEACE TRUST, Tamil Nadu

J. Paul Baskar

1. Introduction

PEACE TRUST is a non-government organisation working among 3,400 child labourers of Dindigul district, since 1984. It has carried out a number of activities for child labour such as Non Formal Education Centres, Child Labour Motivation Camps, Children's Exchange Programme, tours, formation of Child Rights groups, moral development, leadership training, formation of school students association, street play, cultural jathas, legal aid camps, children's library, formation of women, youth, parents, school teachers association for prevention of child labour, anti-child labour campaigns and lobbing advocacy etc, In recent PEACE TRUST focus on rehabilitation of child labourers particularly on organising school enrolment sponsorship programme for spinning mill child workers, The experience of Peace Trust in these rehabilitation programme of spinning mill child worker are briefly presented here.

2. School Enrollment Sponsorship Programme for Cotton Spinning Mill Child Workers

Vedasandur is a taluk in Dindigul district of Tamil Nadu. It is a thickly populated area where immigration and emigration are very common incidents due to drought and unemployment. When there was non-existence of industrial activities, the set up of 52 spinning mills by private people was the first sign of start of any such non-agricultural entrepreneurship in this taluk area. But astonishingly, the evil of child labour emanated along with the emergence of spinning mills in Vedasandur. The growth of this evil knows no bounds when its rate exceeds 25 percent in 300-400 labour population of every mill. The children who are employed in these mills are drawn from those who are in the 11-14 age group. For one shift, they toil 8 hours and earn a wage of Rs. 15 to 20. The nature of work is worst for child workers. They have to walk here and there, in spinning department, which totals upto 30 kilometres per day.

In the campaigns launched by Peace Trust, it was found that, parents send their children to work, in order to fulfil their basic needs and assist the family by bringing in additional income. Hence, the first step in abolishing child labour system, it was realized in our campaigns that the basic and additional needs of families should be fulfilled. The decision was to pull out child labourers from their work place and put them in schools which would be an ideal place for them and in return offer some kind of rewards, mostly in the form of cash, to the parents. From this point of view, Peace Trust started its project "Schooling Enrolment Sponsor ship Programme for Cotton Spinning Mill Child Workers", in 1998.

Identification of Child Labour

A survey on spinning mill child labour was conducted in 243 villages of Vedasandur Taluk, about 630 spinning mill child workers were identified and they were motivated to 'back-to-school' programme. During the door-to-door visit, child workers and parents were explained about the problem of child labour, hazardous occupation, importance of school education and job-oriented courses. The merits of sponsoring, schooling and empowering released child labourers of cotton spinning mills, proved effective.

Selection of Child Labourers

Selection process was organised in four sittings for 417 child workers and their parents. Out of 417 children, 100 child workers were selected for the school enrolment sponsorship programme, on the basis of the following three conditions.

1. The child labour age should be 15 or below.
2. The boy or girl should have worked in the mill for at least 6 month.
3. They should have passed 5th standard in their schools.

Apart from these rules, preference was also given to the child workers who were neglected, victimized, exploited, minority and low-income groups.

Bridge Course Training

In order to change the attitude of the selected child workers from spinning mills to formal schools, a 20-days bridge course was organised in Vedasandur. In this training, all 100 child workers took part actively. Topics like importance of school education and higher studies, problems of child labour, how to manage the school study and family problems, job-oriented courses, Dos and don'ts by children, characters and habits to be followed by child workers in the new school situations were covered under this bridge course training. Apart from these, indoor games, cultural programmes and personal counselling's were given to the children. At end of the bridge course, a foolproof plan was prepared with selected child workers regarding their school re-enrolment, higher studies, attending tuition programme etc.

Enrolment of Child Workers in Formal Schools

The selected 100 children were re-enrolled in seven formal schools located in Vedasandur (Primary School of Girls and Boys High Schools) Poothampatty, Senankottai Sullerumbu, and Devanayackanpatty of Vedasandur Block. Before re-enrolling these children, discussions were made with teachers and headmaster of each school. During these meeting the problem of child labour and importance of re-enrolment of child workers were explained to the school teachers.

Provision of Educational Assistantship

The 100 child labourers under the project were being enrolled at above schools in the same taluk area with all educational assistantships like school admission fees, text books, note books, writing materials, fee for part time vocational training in school, school examination fee, work book fee, travelling allowance to the children from their house to schools, 2 sets of school uniform etc,

Family Cash Stipends

Each parent of ex-child workers is provided with cash stipends of Rs.400/- per month to offset the income lost by the children by working. Such stipends focus on encouraging families to support their children's enrolment in helping the student to attend the school. Under this cash stipend programme, 100 families of ex-child workers are benefited. The main objective of provision of economic incentives for selected 100 poor families is to keep their children in school, to continue their children's education, prevent failure, to stop school dropouts, to provide food to children by parents etc, Now, the parents utilise the stipend for the purpose of purchasing rice, feed to cattle remitting loan taken from money lenders, medical expenses for mother/father, educational expenses for brothers/sisters of ex-child workers. 80 percent of the parents use the stipends for family food.

Arranging Free Bus Pass

In order to avail free bus pass from Government Transport Corporation, we have met managers of Transport Corporation and explained about the "back-to-school" programme for child workers. After a long discussion with them, free bus pass to the ex-child workers were provided. By this effort, about 87 ex-child workers are travelling from their house to schools, free of cost. Peace Trust provides travelling allowance to ex-child workers until issue of free bus pass from the government and for attending holiday special classes.

Tuition Centre For Ex-child Workers

In order to make follow up action to the re-enrolled child workers, to provide supplementary education, to provide opportunity to sit, read and write apart from school timings, a tuition centre was started in the middle of Vedasandur town. The centre functions from 7.30 a.m. to 9.30 a.m. and from 4.00 p.m. - 6.00 p.m. The tuition programme is handled with two qualified teachers; one of them takes the responsibility to cover Mathematics, Science and other covers English, Social Science, and Tamil. In all working days at the above mentioned times, special tuition is held. Weekly educational test is compulsory for the 100 children on all Saturdays.

Children those who have doubts in their subjects, which includes mathematics, grammar, poems, community life, history of India, economic growth, discoveries and use of science, is clarified. Apart from this, topics related to method of writing school examinations, method of scoring high marks, techniques of questions and answers, personality development etc. have also covered. The major activity of the centre is to train the children who were very poor in their education and to facilitate them to score more marks and to get a qualitative and meaningful education.

After this tuition programme, children understood that education will secure their future. Since there is more strength in government schools, child workers re-enrolled by Peace Trust said that they could not follow the teaching in crowded class room (i.e. classes have high strength in each section), besides this tuition centre gave them a good opportunity to revise their subjects continuously. Apart from the school working days, continuous special classes were organised at holidays in tuition centre. It helped the children to memorize the previous class subjects taught in the school. In order to entertain ex-child workers, Peace Trust provides indoor games materials like carom boards, chess boards, music tools, T.V. etc.

Provision of Nutrient Food

One of the most popular incentive strategies is providing free nutrient food to re-enrolled child workers. Under this, everyday all children are provided with milk, egg, biscuits, pulses etc., this provision reduces the costs to parents by providing more nutrient food and helps to ensure that children get the essential energy for learning. The tuition centre provides this nutrients to make the children relive from tiredness.

Health Service and Health Education

Once in two days, health worker visits tuition centre, conducts medical check-ups and distributes medicines free of cost. To prevent diseases of children, they were given health education. Now they are aware about personal hygiene, communicable diseases, first aid, keeping the tuition centre and houses clean etc. Children who suffered from chest pain, eye problem, heart problem and headache are taken to well-equipped hospital, which exist in Madurai for treatment.

Ex-Child Labourers Motivation Camps

To develop managerial capacity, skill and leadership qualities of ex-child workers, to explain job-oriented courses, higher studies, to make them to develop their knowledge, altitude on extra curricular activities and to inculcate the habit of attending school regularly, motivation camps are organized. Topics like child rights, importance of children club, small savings, professional courses, problems of child labour in India, child labour laws and prevention of child labour in cotton spinning mills, are discussed in the camps. The ex-child workers are advised to seek help in clarifying doubts in all subjects, to get moral support within them by educating the weak children. During these camps, the children were encouraged to comprehend their future life. Most of them opted for employment's like computer operator, electrician, office assistant, teachers, doctors, engineer, play writer, village panchayati leader, district civil service officer, defence service personnel etc. Apart from these, cultural programmes like songs, dramas, dances are also conducted in each camp.

Anti-Child Labour Movement by Ex-Child Workers

With ex-child workers, street campaigns were organized in Dindigul town, which dealt with the various issues connected to the new ILO convention on the worst forms of child labour. The ex-child workers and children working in different sectors campaigned the initiative taken by the ILO to eradicate the worst forms of child labour. On the other hand, the street campaigner expressed that the new ILO convention should not serve as a justification for the other forms of child labour. Within the Indian context, where poor children who are involved in labour, cannot have any meaningful programme of education. About 240 child workers including ex-child workers took part in this street campaign programme. Over 5000 bit notices were distributed in Dindigul town and in different parts of Vedasandur taluk through ex-child workers. Nearly 18,000 people become aware of child rights, declaration of worst forms of child labour under new convention of ILO new list of areas to be included in the new convention of ILO, etc.

Parents Motivation Camp Towards Rehabilitation of Child Labour

In order to generate awareness on upgrading ex-child workers, parent's motivation camps are organised every month. Procedures of sending the ex-child workers to schools, helping children to do their home study at night times, method of using the monthly cash stipends, providing nutrient food to ex-child workers, method of upgrading the ex-child workers towards their bright future and evils of child labour were major topics which covered under the parents meetings. At the end of the meetings, the parents were given cash stipends.

Eco-warriors—An Ex-child Workers Environment Club

The 100 students (ex-child workers) are not only availing the advantages of school education and healthy tuition centre, but also a very novel environment training programme exclusively designed for them relying on a set of sophisticated training methods and executed every weekend consecutively for six months in 1999. All 100 children are clubbed into four groups, each group consists 25 members. At week end, one of the four groups is invited and is provided training on environment protection.

Segregating garbage, bio-imagery, travelling to another solar system, finding a tree, creativity and biodiversity, making birds nest, identification of soil erosion and a green pledge were the major topics discussed in the environment training.

To make the ex-child workers socially conscious and futuristically responsible earth citizens group, ECO-WARRIORS--THE NATURE LEADERSHIP FORUM OF CHILDREN was formed. This club has discussed about tree plantation in their schools, maintaining kitchen garden, village sanitation, etc.

Peace Trust will support the ex-child workers up to their 10th standard (S.S.L.C.) and will facilitate them to under go skill training.

2. Alternative Vocational Training for Child Labourers Released from Hazardous Occupation

Child Labour in Tanneries

There were about 2000 child workers in 78 tanneries of Dindigul area, in 1986. While at present only 260 child workers are working in the same industries. For a day's work, they toil from 9.00 a.m. to 6.00.p.m. and earn a wage of Rs. 10 to 15. Being in casual employment, their job is temporary, with no benefits or protection. They have no education and remain as illiterates.

The working condition in tanneries is the worst situation for any child. They have to handle hazardous chemicals without gloves. They even cannot eat proper food because of the odour in the tannery, which would be intolerable. They are usually engaged in removing hair from the leather. This naturally causes Tuberculosis. The worst of all is the drum operation in which children are engaged to get inside a small drum to remove the leather after being soaked in chemicals.

Objectives

The objectives of the alternative vocational training programme are as following:

1. To improve the living conditions of child labourers;
2. To make them stand on their own legs, to help them to learn their own trade; and
3. To enjoy benefits solely by themselves.

Activities

The non-formal Vocational training for child labourers is functioning from April 1996. Till now we have trained 142 children, practical and theoretical training is provided in the following fields:

- Screen printing
- Steel work
- Motor rewinding
- Painting
- Tailoring

- Household wiring
- Refrigerator mechanism
- TV mechanism
- Radio and tape recorder mechanism
- Eliminator assembling.
- Preparation of greeting cards, etc. Because of intensive training, children learn these trades and have started their own units.

They also come to the centre to clarify their doubts. The training is very effective and helps the children to earn and enjoy the profit by themselves. Since they are the masters, the harassment they faced while they worked under some one else is almost negligible. They form their own tactics to improve their trade. They could take their own decisions.

Since the programme directly affects the capitalists, Peace Trust had to face lot of difficulties. Children were not allowed to come to the training centre, parents were threatened and even the suppliers of various goods were forced to stop supplying. But people and the children understood that this programme only helps them to grow and slowly Peace Trust gained momentum. In some of the tanneries, children were not allowed to attend the course, hence children used to come for training on holidays, Sundays and night times as well. We also adjusted the training hours accordingly.

Training materials and equipments were purchased from the nearby towns like Madurai and Trichy. Technical persons and tutors were invited from the Gandhigram Rural Institute, R.V.S. Training centre, Government I.T.I. Dindigul, etc. They assisted us in this endeavour and provided the required technical help and materials means for the programme. By influence of this programme, there are several changes in the status of released child workers. The impact of this project on the children's status is given below:

	Before training	*After training*
1.	Only temporary work was availed.	Permanent employment.
2.	Work was seasonal employment.	Through out the year.
3.	Exploitation and legal rights denied.	Nil exploitation and legal rights preserved.
4.	Working conditions are worse.	Improved working conditions.
5.	More working hours less pay. No share in the profit, stereotype of work.	Desired number of working hours. Profit is enjoyed by self improve or alter techniques, remuneration according to work.
6.	Harassment and ill treat by the employer.	Owner and employer is self so no harassment or ill treat.
7.	Dependency on the employer.	Self-dependency.
8.	No job security.	Secured job is assured.
9.	No power for decision making.	Power to take own decisions.

Thus the programme has more influence on the changes of children's life.

The local NGOs gave a wider publicity and took the message to the masses. They also directed children to the training centre. Some of the local banks have issued small industrial loans, at concession rate of interest, to the trainees to the tune of 10 lakhs. Some of the local shops have procured orders for the products produced by these children. The public also utilize the services of the children trained in this centre to repair their T.V., motor rewinding, house painting, wiring and tape recorders.

17

Overview of Carpet Export Promotion Council

T.S. Chadha

The Carpet Industry in India

Carpet weaving in India is traditional handicraft, passed down from one generation to the next for hundreds of years. A single carpet can take anywhere from a month to a year to weave, depending upon the complexity of the pattern and the number of knots per unit measurement. Carpet weaving is predominately a rural based cottage industry. The carpets are woven on looms installed in cottages, which also serve as the family homes of the loom owners. Children of loom owners are taught the craft of weaving by their parents, in their own homes.

Carpet Export Promotion Council

The Carpet Export Promotion Council was established in 1982 and was registered under Indian Companies Act, 1956. This is the apex body of Indian Carpet Exporters and works on a no profit no loss basis.

The main objective of the Council is to promote sale and exports of the Indian handmade carpets and other floor coverings in the world markets by providing necessary assistance to the carpet manufacturers and exporters. It also strives to initiate steps for the development and growth of the industry.

The Council has achieved tremendous growth in carpet exports through a comprehensive methodology of keeping the Indian exporters abreast of the latest trends and markets worldwide. This is achieved through various means like market surveys, arranging buyer-seller meets, participation in international exhibitions, publicity and providing status reports of overseas buyers.

The Indian carpet industry employs about 2 million people in backward and inaccessible rural areas of the country, where employment opportunities are very limited. In India law prohibits use of child labour in carpet industry. On receiving reports of employment of hired child labour in the carpet industry in eastern Uttar Pradesh, a survey was conducted through a reputed non-governmental agency, by the National Council for Applied Economic Research (NCAER) in 1992, which revealed the incidence of child labour to the extent of 3.6% on hired wage bases. Government took various measures to curb this practice, including prosecution of the offending loom owners and a repeat survey was carried in 1994. The survey revealed that the incidence of child hired on wage basis came down to 2.7% and the awareness of the concerned laws prohibiting child labour has substantially increased.

TABLE 1

Indian Handmade Carpet Industry

Details of Carpet Weaving	
Number of States where carpets are manufactured	15
Largest Concentration of carpet manufacturing state	Uttar Pradesh
Estimated households engaged in weaving	175,000
Estimated Number of Looms	250,000
Number of Looms registered under CEPC	164,000
Estimated number of artisans in carpet weaving	2.5 million

Source: Carpet Export Promotion Council (CEPC).

In response to the widespread media reports about the use of child labour in India, the Council has taken definitive steps to completely eliminate hired child labour from the carpet industry.

The Council is strongly committed to the elimination of illegal child labour in the carpet industry. Towards that end the Council has undertaken significant self-regulating initiatives, one of which is the Code of Conduct for its members for not using child labour. Membership of the Council is mandatory for all carpet exporters as is compliance of the Code of Conduct.

Indian carpet industry took a historic decision to introduce "KALEEN, The Hallmark of Commitment" label for all handmade carpets, druggets, dhuries etc. This label is now being carried by carpets imported from India, as an assurance that no child exploitation has taken place in the manufacture of the product. The user of "KALEEN" label is required to abide by the code of conduct adopted by the Carpet Export Promotion Council for the eradication of child labour.

The Indian carpet industry has also decided to contribute a part of their export earnings w.e.f. 1.4.1995, towards a weavers welfare fund for ensuring:

- Welfare of the weavers community;
- Education of children, with mid-day meals;
- Medical-care of the weavers family; and
- Vocational training of the children with assured stipend.

The Carpet Export Promotion Council's Commitment

The Council stands in firm support of the elimination of illegal child labour in the carpet industry. Towards that end, the Council has undertaken significant self-regulating initiatives, both on its own and in cooperation with the Indian Government. The Council is aggressively tackling the problem. The main elements of the Council's programme for eliminating child labour are as follows:

- Loom Registration Programme.
- Mandatory Code of Conduct.
- Kaleen Label.

1. Loom Registration Programme

The Council launched a major Loom Registration Programme all over India, but most particularly in the state of Uttar Pradesh, where the vast majority of Indian carpets are made. The main elements and objectives of the programme are as follows:

- To create data bank of the names of loom owners (and their photographs) and addresses in order to make monitoring of looms possible.
- Identification of registered looms by displaying of loom registration certificate in the loom shed.
- To obtain an undertaking from each loom owner that he will not employ child labour in violation of the Child Labour (Prohibition and Regulation) Act of 1986 and to inform him of the provisions of the Act including its penal provisions.
- If a loom owner violates the Act then the Council deregisters his loom.
- No exporter is allowed to have carpets made on a deregistered loom (as will be seen from the Code of Conduct below).

2. Code of Conduct

- The Code of Conduct is mandatory for all members of the Council.
- Members undertake that no child labour is used on their premises or in the weaving of their carpets in contravention of the Child Labour (Prohibition and Regulation) Act, 1986.
- Members undertake to get their carpets woven only on registered looms.
- Members prohibited getting carpets woven on de-registered looms.
- In case of violation of the above code on more than two occasions the member will be de-registered from the Council and his membership will be terminated whereby he will not be able to export carpets.

3. The Kaleen Labeling Initiative

The Kaleen label is an assurance to the buyer of the labeled carpet that a contribution has been made from the sales proceeds of the carpet towards the Council's Child Welfare Fund. Kaleen labels are issued only to valid members of the Council who have—

- Made a contribution to the Council's Child Welfare Fund.

- Sworn an affidavit that illegal child labour is not used in the making of his carpets.
- Carpets made only on CEPC registered looms.

The Child Welfare Fund of the Council is used for providing education, mid-day meals, a stipend based on attendance in schools and health care. The CEPC is presently funding 38 schools. The Council has so far issued 10 Lakhs Kaleen labels. 13 schools were provided funds till 1999 in Mirzapur- Bhadhoi carpet weaving belt.

Transparency and Credibility of Kaleen

- Kaleen label is based on an independent transparent and credible inspection mechanism to monitor non-usage of child labour in production of such labeled carpets.
- An independent professional inspection agency has been engaged by the Council to evolve a transparent and credible random inspection mechanism.
- The inspection agency reports to the Council to initiate action against offenders both loom owners and exporters as well inform State Labour Department to initiate action against offenders as per provision of Child Labour (Prohibition & Regulation) Act, 1986.
- The National Level Steering Committee comprising of NGO's, Govt. Officials both Central and State, trade representatives headed by Dev. Commissioner (H) to review the performance of Council's programme.

Overview of CEPC Programme

To ensure the integrity of the Kaleen label and to supervise the implementation of disbursements and programmes under the Child Welfare Fund, a high powered monitoring committee, called the National Steering Committee has been established. The Committee is composed of representatives of the Council, the Government of India, non-governmental organizations, the state governments, the International Labour Organization (ILO), UNICEF and UNDP.

18

Impact of Rehabilitation Programmeson Child Labour

Helen R. Sekar

Policy is the official commitment of a government, normally expressed through the enactment and enforcement of laws. It can exert a powerful influence on national values and public opinion, mobilising financial and institutional resources to a large extent. Policy means a well-defined course of action, adopted and pursued or expedited by a government, political party in power or statesman with authority. The term 'policy' refers to the overall plan of action towards a given goal as distinguished from any specific government action

The special merit of a national policy lies in the fact that it articulates societal objectives and commitment and, if pursued faithfully, provides a coherent framework for an associated programme of action. Such a national policy and programme of action can stand on its own or comprise part of a more comprehensive policy; in either case a complete and effective national policy and programme of action generally contains at least the elements such as a definition of national objectives; a description of the nature and context of the problem; identification and description of the priority target groups; a description of the intervention approaches to be used and the designation of the institutional actors to be involved

(2) Government policy, requires public backing and the involvement of the non-governmental sector.

A clear national policy against the exploitation of children is the fundamental basis and point of significance for governmental action to combat child labour. The phenomenon of child labour, which has spread throughout the world, is a glaring example of the fundamental violation of the rights of a child. The extent of violation of children's rights and the ever increasing cases of child abuse, not only depict the gross indifference of the society, at large, towards this sensitive issue, but also calls for an effective strategy of governance, based on a greater concern for children facing the onslaught of deprivation. For large number of children work in an ordeal, a source of suffering and exploitation.

A policy on child labour is a public commitment to work towards the elimination of child labour, setting out objectives and priorities, coupled with the resource provision to ensure implementation. Child Labour Policy is also reflected in both legislation and administrative regulations the goal of public policy on child labour in India is to provide increased protection to working children and gradually reducing the incidence of child labour. The policy implication may be measured in two different ways:

(i) through an intimate link between child labour and the employment and income status of households. Here the provision of schemes that generate and enhance employment and income among the adult workers is a necessary condition for the reduction of child labour and
(ii) through a link between child labour and provision of schooling. The vital determinants here are the need to expand educational facilities with improved quality of curriculum and teaching methods, backed up with a programme of nutrition.

The specific aim of this paper is to examine the existing inputs in the policy framework and the programmes of action for dealing with the issue of child labour. Provisions in the Indian Constitution have ensured the establishment of a Welfare State in India. These have been further reinforced and strengthened in subsequent policies of the government. The philosophy of welfare State is very much reflected in the chapter on Directive Principles of State Policy of the Constitution. By incorporating the term 'socialist' in the preamble to the Indian Constitution, the objective of a Welfare State has been reinforced.

In so far as policy measures promoting a welfare state is concerned, the state has always played a pre-dominant role in providing for health, education and safety nets. Several policies have been formulated in this respect. The State in India is committed to provide for the welfare of children, to prevent their exploitation, and to prohibit and regulate the employment of children below a certain age. This commitment arises from certain constitutional provisions, India's ratification of the several ILO Conventions, its participation in the UN Declaration of the Rights of the Child, enactment of a number of statutes on the subject of child labour and in other areas connected with child welfare, and from the fact that India is a welfare state.

The Constitution-makers were conscious of the need for the special care of children. The 'Significant provision under Article 23 of the Constitution of India to ensure that no traffic in human beings and other forms of forced labour occurs, the provision of Article 24 states that no child shall be employed in any factory or mine or engaged in other hazardous employment; all the provisions of Article 39 directing the State to form policies towards securing that children are not abused or exploited, and are given opportunities and the provision of Article 45 requiring the state to endeavour to provide free and compulsory education for all children till the age of 14 years, is a clear indication that the underlying dimensions of the existence of child labour had been correctly diagnosed at the time of the framing of the Constitution.

The task of translating these constitutional provisions into appropriate state mechanisms for addressing the problem of child labour was initiated once the magnitude and dimensions of the problems were seen to have overtaken the existing legal provisions. A National Policy on Child Labour and a comprehensive central legislation prohibiting or regulating child labour were the two underpinnings of the renewed efforts to address the issue and both were formulated in the second half of the eighties.

The first comprehensive attempt towards a national policy was taken in 1987 with the adaptation of the National Policy on Child Labour. It had two main objectives. The long-term objective was to eradicate child labour and protect all children from exploitation. The short-term objective was to improve the conditions of work, nutrition and health-related factors of child labourers.

The National Child Labour Policy had identified a three-pronged action plan to realise these objectives namely: the legislative action plan to ensure effective implementation of the existing laws related to child labour; the focussing of general development programmes for benefiting child labour wherever possible (this entailed ensuring the implementation of programmes concerning education, health, nutrition and anti-poverty measures); and a project based plan of action in areas of high concentration of child labour engaged in wage and quasi-wage employments.

In pursuance of the National Child Labour Policy, National Child Labour Projects were started in child labour endemic districts of the country in 1988-89. The National Child Labour Policy envisages focussing of different development and welfare programmes for the benefit of working children. In the National Child Labour Project areas, an integration of such programmes was attempted. The activities targeted to be taken up in these projects were: stepping up enforcement of child labour laws; non-formal education; adult education; income and employment generation; operation of special schools; raising public awareness; and survey and evaluation.

By the end of 1994, 12 child labour projects were sanctioned in the states of Andhra Pradesh (Jaggampet and Markapur), Bihar (Garhwa), Madhya Pradesh (Mandsaur), Maharashtra (Thane), Orissa (Sambalpur), Rajasthan (Jaipur), Tamilnadu (Sivakasi), and Uttar Pradesh (Varanasi-Mirzapur-Bhadohi, Moradabad, Aligarh and Firozabad).

A major programme was subsequently announced on 15th August 1994 for the withdrawal and rehabilitation of an estimated two million children working in hazardous occupations. In pursuance of the announcement, a number of child labour projects were sanctioned for coverage of more children under the National Child Labour Projects. By the end of 1995-96, a total of 76 projects had been sanctioned for coverage of 1.5 lakh children through 2500 special schools. As per the latest available information, only 1.05 lakh children have been enrolled in 1800 special schools.

Establishment and running of the special schools is the major activity under the National Child Labour Project at the ground level. The special schools provide non-formal education, vocational training, supplementary nutrition, stipend, health care, etc. to children withdrawn from employment. These children are put in special schools for three years. After completion of three years in special schools, children are expected either to join the mainstream formal education or take up job or self employment venture. As per the existing scheme of the National Child Labour Project, the vocational component of the special schools is required to be imparted along with the formal education. On the basis of field studies and secondary data, an attempt has been made to examine the effectiveness of the National Child Labour Project. In Burdwan district, West Bengal, 36 special schools were operational out of 39 schools sanctioned in which 1850 children were enrolled. Of these 1108, were male and 752 were female. The children in the age group of 9-11 years numbered 858 and that in 12-14 years was 992. Prior to joining the special schools, these children were employed in bidi making, auto industry, hotel/restaurant, construction, weaving, chemical industry, cycle repairs etc,.

Sholapur in Maharashtra, was the first district to start special schools for child labour. In this district, child labour was concentrated in power looms, bidi making and construction. Here 22 special schools were operational accommodating 1100 boys and girls. The project society in the district had a multidisciplinary approach and was adopting the strategy of joyful learning in schools. The project also laid emphasis on convergence of services, for which it had partnership with academic institutions and NGOs.

In Aligarh district of Uttar Pradesh, 10 schools were functional under the National Child Labour Project (NCLP). Environment building and awareness generation through slides, rallies, meetings and discussions were important components of this project society.

Forty special schools were opened in different blocks and municipalities of North 24 Parganas district in West Bengal. In the special schools there were 80 per cent attendance in rural areas and about 60-80 per cent in the urban areas. Awareness generation programmes have been taken up through Panchayati Raj bodies and municipalities. It was reported that teachers faced problems because of the large variation in the age of students.

Under the NCLP, forty special schools were sanctioned for 2000 children in Coimbatore district, Tamilnadu. Along with setting up of schools, an attempt had been made to bring about attitudinal change among families by organising the mothers of child labourers into small groups namely 'Self-help Women Groups'. These groups were functioning as 'social pressure groups ' and 'vehicles of change' and also undertaking the responsibility of sending the children of the members to schools.

In Firozabad district of Uttar Pradesh, 40 special schools had been sanctioned under the NCLP in which total 3332-child labourers were enrolled. In addition to these children, 2246-child labourer were enrolled in primary schools and other informal centres running under the education department of the state government. A special enrolment drive had been launched in this district and 6137-child labourer were identified and enrolled in primary schools, special schools and informal education centres. There was a need to enrol 8000 to 10000 identified child labourer for which 30 additional special schools were needed. Non-governmental organisations were also playing a significant role in managing the child labour schools in Firozabad. Ten special schools of 150-child labourer each were being managed by the District Council of Child Welfare. In addition, eight special schools with an enrolment of 487-child labourer were run by three different voluntary organisations.

Twenty special schools had been opened in Jaipur district, Rajasthan, covering 1000 children, with the programme of mid-day meal, free books and regular health checkups. The National Council of Education Research and Training (NCERT) teaching and learning materials were being followed. Awareness generation was being imparted through poster competition, debates, essay competition, etc.

In Kalahandi district, Orissa, out of a total of 2,35,000 families, 2,05,000 were below the poverty line. It is viewed in this district that child labour is, a dire, unalterable necessity of life and a child has to work in order to meet his daily food requirements. Thirty-six special schools had been set up at different places in Kalahandi district. These schools had 90 per cent retention rate, since the method of joyful learning was being followed in schools. Vocational skills were also imparted in these schools, which could be of immediate use for the economic sustenance of children. Every school had a mothers' committee meeting once a week. Many families were getting support from programmes like Integrated Rural Development Programme (IRDP) and Indira Awas Yojana.

Forty special school buildings had been constructed in Malkangiri district, Orissa. Not all the schools were functional there. In the schools that were functional, the State Council of Education

Research and Training (SCERT) course material had been adopted. Awareness generation programme had been launched in which National Social Service volunteers were involved. Despite geographical and topographical disadvantages and adverse demographic features, social mobilisation of parents, teachers and students towards elimination of child labour problem was made possible through effective implementation of various programmes by the project society

Garwa is a small district situated at the tri-junction of Bihar, Uttar Pradesh and Madhya Pradesh. The problem of child labour in this district is related to poverty, high levels of illiteracy, crop failure for a few years and perennial drought. Four special schools had been opened in this district. Out of 3800 child labourer that had been identified as working in carpet looms, 225 children were enrolled in special schools. As far as targeting child labour families with developmental programmes were concerned, very little had been done so far.

In Surat district, Gujarat, 4934 child labourer had been identified. These children were working in the diamond cutting industry. Out of 4934 child labourer, 978 had been enrolled in 18 special schools. The teaching technique in these schools was absolutely non-formal, based on the concept of joyful learning. Vocational training was given in seven different trades. Several awareness generation programmes had been conducted on the issue of child labour.

In Udaipur district, Rajasthan, 2333 child labourer had been identified. All these children were working in the construction industry. In the 34 special schools that were functional, non-formal education system had been adopted. Vocational training was at a very early stage of implementation. Public awareness on the issue of child labour had been generated through pamphlets, cinema slides, films, posters and hoardings.

Mandsaur, a district in the state of Madhya Pradesh is known for its slate pencil industry. The NCLP was started in Mandsaur in the year 1988. Out of 1357 child labour identified from the slate pencil industry, 500 children were studying in special schools. Eight special schools had been set up in the district. One of the components of the special schools was vocational training. Training was being imparted in the following areas: book binding, soap making, electrical wiring, chair making and handicrafts. Though the vocational training had proved successful in general, certain vocations like handicrafts and soap making were not popular as they were not economically viable. Preference was given to electrical wiring. However, children had not been able to use their skills in this area, as they were not given tool kits, nor were they provided with the loan to buy the same. Although the special schools were for both boys and girls, girls generally dropped out when they attained puberty, thereby limiting the impact of the project. Stricter enforcement of child labour legislation was one of the most noticeable features of the NCLP in this district. The child labour laws were being enforced effectively with regular and repeated inspections. This had been possible because of the Joint Enforcement Committee, which was set up in the district. This Committee comprised of the Collector of the district, labour department officials and the Project Director.

From the above review of the functioning of various programmes under the NCLP, it appears that the special schools component of the programme package has been reasonably successful. However, in the area of awareness generation, very little had been achieved and the funds released remained largely unused. The operationalisation of the special schools programme has been somewhat sketchy and the approach towards the programme has been sceptical. To start with, there was confusion on which type of children were to be admitted in the special schools. Interestingly, in some states like Bihar, Uttar Pradesh and Madhya Pradesh, many children going to the corporation schools shifted to these special schools for the simple reason that stipend was to be given to each child enrolled in the special schools. This was absolutely contrary to the basic objectives of the special schools programme.

Another major flaw in the special schools programme relate to the development of curricula or teaching material for students. The age heterogeneity factor has created obstacle in evolving a fool-proof teaching aid, catering to the needs of children ranging in the age group of 5-14 years. The development of course content in the special schools programme is still, in a stage of experimentation. It is desirable to evolve and Minimum Levels of Learning (MLL) strategy and segregate children on the basis of age group. It is also necessary to redefine the whole admission criteria to special schools and put it on some reasonable footing based on ground realities. Necessary checks should be made to ensure that only the intended target group benefits.

Running of special schools under the NCLP is very cost intensive, since the cost involved per child is about Rs.4000, whereas in the formal schools the cost per child is only Rs. 1000. It is cost intensive as it is integrated in character and combines the elements of education, nutrition, health and vocational skill training. Working children are different from normal children and are placed in a situation of acute social disadvantage. Dealing with working children means dealing with a multi-age, multi-level and multi-skilled target group who cannot be put into a uniform basket. They are clearly in need of specialised preferential treatment. The teachers in these special schools were not in a position to provide them the healing touch, which could mitigate their traumatised mental state. Special orientation, re-orientation and training are necessary for these teachers. Most of the special schools were not functioning as per norms. The teachers were not being recruited properly, there was no involvement of the community in the process of selection and no proper training was being imparted to the teachers. The curriculum, course content and textual materials used in special schools did not correspond to the pedagogic and functional needs of the working children.

One of the important elements of the strategy for the prevention and elimination of child labour under the NCLP is awareness generation for which a sum of Rs. 5 lakhs has been earmarked for each of the 133 child labour endemic districts in the country. Certain myths about child labour can only be removed through spreading knowledge about the evils of child labour, exploitation and abuse of working children and the impact of health hazards on the physical and mental growth of a child. Awareness generation activities carried out under the NCLP had a very limited impact.

Child labour exists across the vast geographical stretch of India is characterised by wide socio-economic variations, existence of a variety of languages, customs, traditions, etc. This calls for different strategies for awareness generation campaign for sensitising people at the grass roots level, who would ultimately be instrumental in implementing schemes for the elimination of child labour. Media can play a very important role in supporting social mobilisation efforts for the elimination of child labour. It is important that efforts are made for formulating a comprehensive multimedia strategy, which would then be translated into media action in terms of media services and product and is implemented in a concerted, planned and sequential manner to cover various groups of people at different level, namely district, state and national level. The media strategy thus developed should be used both by the government and mass media so that appropriate messages on prevalence and evils of child labour are conveyed to all.

Income and employment generating schemes are considered to be fundamental to achieving a reduction in the incidence of child labour. The assumption is that if the economic status of the family improves, there will be less need for child to work. It is therefore planned that the activities currently carried out within the framework of the IRDP, NREP and RLEGP in the project areas be stepped up.

In terms of the NCLP, the emphasis on general development programme has remained unimplemented. The bureaucratic nature of the government operations, comes in the way of delivering their services effectively. Recognizing the need for a flexible approach, the government has been increasingly interested in involving voluntary agencies. But this solution also had problems. Many of the voluntary agencies were located in urban or town areas and tended to work around these areas. The resources allotted to them therefore did not reach the rural areas where the magnitude of child labour was more pronounced. Rural areas where voluntary organisations do not operate got lesser or no share of the benefits of the programme.

In the income generation programme, minimum wages are not at par with the wages in the organised sector and Central and State governments. The Minimum Wages Act does not provide guidelines for fixing wages. The revision of minimum wages is not being done regularly. Therefore, the income levels are very low. The prevalence of child labour is largely due to low family income.

Implementing agencies of child labour programmes were neither aware of all income generation programmes nor were they conscious about how this could be utilised. The beneficiaries too also lacked knowledge and awareness to avail of these programmes,

The ultimate objective of development, of any society, is to improve the quality of life of the majority of its people and one of the determinants of quality of life is the state of health and nutrition. NCLP has extended the development of health care of children to those areas where child labour is prevalent, irrespective of whether they are in primary school, or at work. It has felt the need for persuading the state governments to extend the coverage of school health services programme to child labour and to maintain the persuasion so that all children are covered by regular health inspections and treatment/referral services and health screening at non-formal education centres are arranged.

In Sivakasi, 18 per cent of the parents of child labour interviewed, reported to have utilised the facilities at primary health centres and sub-centres. The utilisation of government district hospitals and ESI hospitals was reported by 28 per cent of the parents. Almost all of them were aware of the existence of government hospitals or PHCs in their area or nearby area. About 80 per cent of them went to private medical practitioners. The reasons for non-use of government health services were geographical location non-availability of medicines and improper behaviour of the MC staff. The reasons adduced for utilising government health services were that the services were free or cheap. The very poor who could not afford private health services were using the free government out patient services.

Voluntary organisations are reportedly more successful in providing health care services to the poor in general and child labour families in particular. NGO experiences, by and large, showed that they were able to improve health status considerably at the current level of socio economic development. Factors contributing to their success seemed to be women health workers at village level, accessible medical facility, high community participation and integration with some developmental activities. NGO programmes reported better utilisation and higher impact on health indicators compared to the government programmes.

With regard to nutrition, the National Child Labour Policy states that Department of Women and Child Development have an on going programme for women and children i.e. Integrated Child Development Services, which are approved on the basis of the proposals by the state government and non-governmental organisations. While it will not be possible to earmark funds specifically for child labour, proposals from state government and non-governmental organisations in child labour areas will be funded on a priority basis, if necessary, the rules could be relaxed to consider proposals from the organisation to be set up for taking up welfare measures for child labour also. For millions of child labour families, according to macro-level data, incomes were too low to provide dietary adequacy at the given food prices. The nutrition status as measured by average heights and weights by age is also lesser for child labour compared to other children because of the combination of malnutrition and hazardous working conditions.

Available data suggests that despite the launching of National Child Labour Project, the food consumption and nutrition intake of the child labour families had remained either the same or have declined in some places. Though the incidence of severe malnutrition in the population had declined among working children and their families overall it did not seem to have reduced.

Unlike the health programme, the nutrition programmes were specifically directed towards the poor and the disadvantaged groups in the community. Poverty eradication was seen as a necessary condition for better nutrition status. The Tamil Nadu Noon Meal Programme run by the Government is one of the most extensive supplementary feeding programme currently undertaken in any developing country using its own resources. It covers children between 2 and 14 years of age in the State of Tamilnadu. The objective of this programme is, to feed the children, less than 14 years of age, belonging to the poor families, one wholesome meal per day. In addition, children receive health and nutrition services, one major feature of this programme is the employment of thousands of poor women. For this reason, it is also considered an anti-poverty programme.

Though the mid-day meal programme under the NCLP has had a positive impact on the nutritional status of children attending the school and child labour but children of the poorest of the poor do not seem to have benefited as much. This could be because lesser number of children from the child labour families attends school regularly.

The Integrated Child Development Services (ICDS) scheme was initiated in 1975-76. Its major objectives were to reduce malnutrition, morbidity and mortality among children under the age of 6 years, provide the conditions necessary for their psychosocial development and enhance the ability of mothers to take care of their children. To achieve these goals a package of services consisting of supplementary feeding, immunisation, health check-up, referral services, nutrition and health education were offered.

Interviews with ICDS workers in the study area reveal that though children in the ICDS areas receive immunisation and nutrition services, the scheme was not successful in reaching the poor residing in isolated areas. It was reported that very poor families and more so the child labour families were inhibited by the fact that their children did not have proper clothing for attending the Anganwadis. Also, children who were neither going to school nor work were required at home to look after their younger siblings. One major criticism against this programme is that a lot of children who come for feeding are not in dire need of nutritional supplements. Though they generally come from poor families they do not belong to the poorest families or child labour families.

Some of the nutrition programmes run by the non-governmental agencies have achieved remarkable success by working on the premise that desirable improvement in the nutritional status can be brought about only through a multi-pronged attack on all its major attributes.

Experience from both the government and non-government programmes showed that nutritional interventions were more effective when they were a part of community development efforts with complementary measures to reduce poverty and hunger. NGO experiences reveal that health was not a priority felt-need of the poor; rather their priority was water or employment depending upon their situation. Similarly priority was given to programmes related to feeding and not to the attainment of nutritional standards. Therefore action research is needed about how health and nutrition can be made an integral part of poverty alleviation and elimination of child labour.

Being a welfare State, it is not surprising to see the myriad welfare measures that the Government of India has initiated towards realising the objectives of the National Child Labour Policy. However, the impact has not so far been very significant. One of the important reasons for the inadequate impact is that enforcement of laws and implementation of programmes has not been adequately monitored. The present levels of monitoring have not provided a meaningful base for improving policy action and corrective measures. Establishment of a meaningful monitoring system and getting sustained feedback thereof would alone achieve the objective of weaning children out of work.

The welfare measures are seldom addressed directly to children. Any benefit which accrues to the children is by virtue of their being a part of a large unit of their family. Even the schemes to ameliorate the conditions of child labourers do not address the root causes behind the child labour issue. While the government has been able to implement the NCLP successfully in certain areas, it has been unsuccessful in most of the project areas. This may be due to lack of understanding of area specific socio-economic realities. No two regions have similar socio-economic conditions. In fact no two situations of child labour are similar. One cannot, therefore, formulate universal strategy for eliminating child labour.

REFERENCES

Balwant Singh, *Labour Policy and Administration* (New Delhi: M.D Publications, 1996), p. 9.

Helen R. Sekar, *Girl Child Labour in the Match Industry of Sivakasi: No Light in Their Life* (Noida : NRCCL, V.V. Giri National Labour Institute, 1993).

Targeting the Intolerable (Geneva: ILO, 1996), p. 100.

Implementation on National Child Labour Projects (Noida NRCCL, V.V. Giri National Labour Institute, 1997).

Helen R. Sekar, *Child Labour Legislation in India: A Study in Retrospect and Prospect* (Noida: NRCCL, V.V. Giri National Labour Institute, 1997).

19

Child Labour Rehabilitation in India: A Case Study of Mirzapur-Bhadhoi Carpet Weaving Belt

Bupinder Zutshi

Introduction

The global perspective of child labour as a human right violation and social development issue has given way to the convention that children have rights, the same full spectrum of rights as adults. This convention, expressed as the convention of the Rights of the child, entered into international law on, 2nd September 1990, nine months after the convention's adoption by the United Nations General Assembly. The convention has been ratified by majority of countries, including India.[1] The other important international instruments on child labour being the ILO's Minimum Age Convention No. 138 and the ILO convention No. 182 on the Elimination of the Worst Forms of Child Labour. Convention No. 138 regulates work conditions and specifies the minimum age for entering into workforce, whereas Convention No. 182 prohibits the children up to 17 years of age in specified work processes which are harmful to the their life and limb, their health, their psyche and their total development. However both the Conventions No. 138 and 182 are yet to be ratified by India and pressure is being applied to ratify both the conventions at the earliest. Under the UN Conventions on Rights of the Child, the country is obliged in law to undertake all appropriate measures to assist parents and other responsible parties in fulfilling their obligations to children (Article 6, 12, 18, 24, 27, 28, 31, 32 of the Rights of Child). The process of implementing the conventions is still in its early stages and requires preparation of appropriate and adequate conditions for its full implementation.

According to revised estimates as assessed by the International Labour Organization (ILO), Bureau of Statistics, the number of working children in the world between the ages of 5 and 14 years is at least 120 million. India with a population of more than 1 billion in 2000 A.D., has the largest population of these working children in the world.[2] The issues of addressing child labour took a pronounced tone in India during the last two decades as the ILO bracketed India along with other countries for the sheer magnitude of this problem. It necessitated certain fundamental changes in national laws, plans, policies and practices to bring them into line with the principles of the Conventions on the Right of the Child.

The Children of the Loom—a film made by British Broadcasting Corporation (BBC), on children in Mirzapur- Bhadhoi carpet weaving belt, who were found to be bonded labourers, has prompted many child welfare organizations in Europe and America to pressurize the importers not to buy Indian products, unless the manufacturers took significant steps to humanize child labour, who are working in these processes. This has resulted in a sharp decline of carpet and other export products made by children from India.

Senator Harkin's proposed child labour Deterrence Bill, which was introduced in the United States (US) legislature on 5th August 1992 states, "US ought not to import any item, from any country, that is made by child labour."[3] This has created alarm bells for Government of India and other exporters to urgently address the issues of child labour. German carpet importers have also threatened to boycott Indian hand knotted carpets, until they are satisfied that no child labour has been involved in its manufacturing.

The issue of child labour has generated renewed interest, because of the new economic policy formulated is in line with the Structural Adjustment Programme, which hopes to put the country on the global market economy. These sweeping economic reforms aim to promote exports and offer incentives to foreign investors. The reforms have affected cuts in the expenditure on health, education, food subsides and on social services, the poor need all these for their basic survival. Thus, the real cost of adjustment is likely to be paid by the poor and by their children, who would be compelled to work at the lower wages provided for the work. The logic of globalisation of the economy has now become a reality in the form of the World Trade Organisation (WTO), which is even eyeing to take over the social aspects in international cooperation through the proposed social clauses. Soaring inflation and massive retrenchment from the industrial sector, especially of women and unskilled labour, unprecedented displacement of the poor peasantry from land and from the traditional occupations have been the order of the day. This has contributed significantly to the large scale presence of child labour in manufacturing process that are harmful to their physical and mental development.

The large-scale presence of working children is a symptom of the disease that is widespread due to exploitative structure, lopsided development and iniquitous resource ownership. Other parameters contributing to its presence in India are, rampant unemployment, rapid urbanization, fast population growth, extreme poverty, increasing disparities in wealth, cut backs in government social and educational budgets, high level of child abuse by the parents/ society and a breakdown of traditional family and community structures.[4] Human migrations from rural to urban areas have contributed significantly to a substantial increase in the number of working children. These migrants shift to cities in search of higher income and secure employments. However, they are able to secure jobs mostly in the unorganised or semi-organized low-paid sector. Consequently, children are forced to earn livelihood for themselves and also support their families.

Child labour has emerged as an increasingly important issue in the national context, reflecting heightened sensitivity to the problem at all levels within the country, especially after the Supreme Court directions on child labour in December 1996. The issue has become more prominent with the growing activism of the human right wings especially the National Human Rights Commission of India.

In this background, strong sentiments are being evoked because of large-scale employment of child labour in general and their presence in hazardous industries particularly in India. There is helplessness of the industrialists, legislative machinery and the social activists to reach a broad agreement for opposing this abominable practice. Completing the paradox is the virtual exclusion of parents and the working children from the whole debate, as well as divergent approaches of the intellectuals, while addressing to this problem.[5] The Supreme Court in its directions in 1996, has ordered for immediate identification of children in hazardous occupations and their subsequent rehabilitation. The directions has pressurised the government to conduct a census of children working in hazardous occupation. However, the survey results indicates under reporting in the identification of children in the hazardous occupations, as the number of identified children were much less, contrary to the estimates given by several studies and NGOs.

Education and Child Labour

Child labour is really the problem of lack of child education and adult unemployment. These two, are perhaps, the most crucial links in a vicious circle. Child labour virtually becomes not only co-terminus with educational deprivation, but also co-terminus with the death of a succeeding generation. The framers of the Indian constitution consciously incorporated relevant provisions in the Constitution like (Article 45) which advocates compulsory universal elementary education up to 14 years of age for all children.[6] However the basic goal of compulsory education up to the age of 14 years has yet to be achieved owing to lack of political commitment and will. The proposal of recognizing elementary education as a 'fundamental right' is now being recognized through the proposed 93rd constitutional amendment, which has already been passed by the lower house in 2001. It is hoped that the amendment will be adopted in the upper house also, in the near future. But at present the schooling system is nowhere near to provide education of decent quality to every child[7]. Contrary to the claims by education department, the primary school in India is inaccessible for a significant proportion of the rural population because of a variety of reasons.[8] Moreover, along with ineffective teaching, the schools remain closed for majority of time, due to poor supervision and management.[9] Perhaps due to these reasons elementary education has not been made compulsory in India, whereas several developing countries have gone ahead and made primary education compulsory long before achieving economic development.[10] Thus complete withdrawal of child labour from the work is difficult to attain in the short run unless immediate measures are taken for making child education compulsory.

Non-Formal Education—Significance

A comprehensive strategy to combat child labour must begin with high quality schools and relevant educational programs. The families should be willing to send their children for education to these schools. Primary education system in its present form is unacceptable, unrealistic, and unreachable to the children of poor, downtrodden and rural families. It is established that, work can keep children away from school. At the same time, poor quality of education, often causes children to drop-out/'push-out'[11] of schools and start working at an early age. Our results testify that drop- out rates in Mirzapur-Bhadohi carpet belt is very high as out of 100 children enrolled in primary schools, 33 reach up to primary level, 8 reach up to middle level and only 1 child reaches up to high school level. Prof. Yash Pal, Chairman of National Advisory Committee in 1993, states joy-less learning as a major problem for 'push-outs'.

> "Both the teacher and the child have lost the sense of joy in being involved with educational process. Teaching and learning . . . to the majority of our school going children are made to view at school as a boring, even unpleasant and bitter experience. They are daily socialized to look upon education as mainly a process of preparing for examination, no other motivation seems to have any legitimacy."

If schools are to attract and retain children, their courses have to be seen as relevant by both parents and children. One prerequisite of a successful state education program is that it links the lessons taught to community life. Schools have to adapt to children's circumstances. The annual calendar and daily time-table of a school must be adjusted according to the seasonal farming calendar in the area.[12] Schools also have to move towards children particularly in far-flung and isolated rural areas, so that education is brought within easy walking distances. A simplified curriculum and locally produced learning materials must be evolved. Teachers with modest formal education have proven to be effective, when given concerted practical training and frequent in-service upgrades. Rigid traditional teaching methods must give way to child centered approaches. The National Policy of Education, 1986, has reemphasized that the academic program and school activities should be built around the child and that the emphasis should be shifted from mere enrollment to retention and to the quality of education.[13]

The sheer size of the population, non-availability of government school in rural areas and in-operational school education has lead to a growing realization among the people and policy and plan makers, that Non-formal Education (NFE) is the best alternative to inculcate educational awareness in the isolated, underdeveloped areas. The most significant step in this direction was the adoption of National Policy of Education (NPE-1986) and National Policy of Child Labour (NPCL-1987). Both these policies aimed at successfully rehabilitating child labour released from hazardous employment and to reduce the incidence of child labour progressively. The opening of the special school for imparting NFE and vocational training was the major recommendation of the two policies.

It is generally admitted that government primary schools are not really appropriate to the needs of many rural children. The existing program of education does not attract girls in the age group of 6-14. On the contrary, NFE models have proved their efficacy in reaching to the poor and down trodden sections of the society. It has all the elements, which in the opinion of the policy makers constitute a "good" program, and at the same time it is cost effective. It's intended clientele would come from children of weaker section like ST/SC/ hilly areas/tribal areas/urban slums/economically backward rural areas. However after initial NFE all the children must be streamlined into formal system. The focus is to serve under privileged sections of the community, which remain unserved by the existing government school system. Anil Bordia[14] urged "that expenditure on improving the facilities in government primary school, would do little to the poor, who dropout, where as the system of NFE is targeted to meet the needs of working children."

Almost all attempts to bring education to working children and children released from hazardous occupations, have been through non-formal education programs, independent of the education system. Mirzapur-Bhadohi carpet belt was identified as one of the project based plan of action by NPCL-1987. Under this plan of action provision of non-formal education, vocational training, supplementary nutrition, and stipend for children released from prohibited employments was stipulated. The actual implementations were carried out by local non-governmental organizations. The successful literacy campaign has generally been found to be executed by NGO's, as they enjoy an element of enlightened voluntarism close to grass root reality with a requisite organizational strength.

Government Initiatives

Sensing the magnitude and momentum generated on the child labour issues, governmental of India, passed several legislative measures to prohibit or improve the working conditions of child labour (Child Labour Act-1986). The legislation has started bearing fruits, but the situation demands strict enforcement along with creating conducive conditions for promoting and providing education services for the working children and children released from various hazardous occupations. The government realised that mere legislation will not be sufficient hence, it initiated several action oriented programmes, to withdraw children from hazardous work, and mainly to prevent them from entering into labour markets again. Project based action plan, in the areas of high concentration of child labour have been introduced and implemented under the action plan of National Child Labour Projects (NCLP). Since the released children from hazardous occupations are of older age groups, hence their immediate integration with formal schools are considered inappropriate unless they were provided orientation course to reach up to the level of formal schools. These orientation courses are designed through Non-formal Education (NFE).

National Policy of Education, 1986 (NPE) proposed Non-formal education schools for the released child labour from hazardous industries and for the working children to provide them need based education under the NCLP programme. 4,90,000 Non-Formal Education (NFE) centres were proposed under the programme, which will supplement the formal education system.[15] Since the central feature of the implementation of the strategy for non-formal education is based on micro-level and area specific and population specific planning, NFE schools for child labour were required to be set up with the involvement of voluntary agencies and Panchayati Raj institutions. The institutions must be capable of running Non-Formal Education Centres, to cater to the needs of the released child labour from hazardous occupations or to the children who may attend these centres during work hours or holidays. A special attention is required to attract and retain working girl children to these NFE schools.

The aim of such Non-Formal Education Centres, is to educate children up to class V level through an accelerated 3 years educational package. The method of teaching should be appropriately designed, so that the children after the 3 years of Non-formal Education will be integrated into formal schools in class VI. Along with the Non-formal Education, the scheme envisaged, vocational training, imparting of age-appropriate craft and pre-vocational training. The vocational skills imparted should be based on the available local resources and market forces of the area, so that children unable to join formal schools after 14 years of age could start their own occupations. Other benefits include supplementary nutrition diet, regular health care and stipend. It also envisaged extension of benefits of the other State Central Government programmes like; healthcare, poverty alleviation schemes and nutritional diet etc; for these school children and their families by the district administration as far as possible.

Government of India has implemented NCLP in 100 districts of the country covering the states of Andhra Pradesh (22 districts), Bihar (8 districts), Karnataka (3 districts), Madhya Pradesh (7 districts), Maharastra (2 districts), Orissa (18 districts), Punjab (1 district), Rajasthan (5 districts), Tamil Nadu (9 districts), Uttar Pradesh (11 districts), and West Bengal (7 districts).[16]

The National Human Rights Commission of India (NHRC) has taken a proactive role to monitor the NCLP programme in the project areas after the Supreme Court directions. Several visits by the Special Rapporteur and other esteemed members of the NHRC in the identified project areas have helped to improve the conditions of NCLP schools. The visits have also given a strong message to the employers of the children that strict measures would be initiated against them, if the Child Labour Act, 1986 and Bonded Labour Act is violated in its true spirit. The message has gone loud and clear in the project areas and significant positive changes is being witnessed towards the attitude of the employers for employing children in the hazardous occupations.

Voluntary Sector Initiatives

To supplement government initiatives, several national and international donor agencies got deeply involved in the elimination of child labour and protecting the working children from exploitation and abuse. Several NFE schools were started in the Mirzapur - Bhadhoi carpet belt of Uttar Pradesh and Bihar. The NFE centres were sponsored by Ministry of Labour, Government of India under International Program of Elimination of Child Labour (IPEC) and Child Labour Action Support Program (CLASP) of International Labour Organization (ILO). In addition to government sponsored NFE centres, other NFE centres were started by Project Mala, CREDA, REHA Consortium, CRY, UNICEF and other local based NGOs. By 1995-96 a large number of NFE schools were in operation in Mizapur-Bhadhoi carpet belt, providing NFE to the released children from carpet weaving.

Objectives of the Study

The objective of the present study is to examine the functioning of the NFE special schools undertaken by the Project Societies/NGOs in the carpet weaving belt of Mirzapur- Bhadhoi in Uttar Pradesh state. The study aims to evaluate the NFE schools, examine their impact in reducing child labour and study the Community response and acceptance towards the NFE special school activities related to education and rehabilitation of children. The results of the study would be extremely useful for future planning of non-formal education to eradicate child labour in carpet weaving. The results of the study would provide valuable inputs for suggesting recommendations to improve the NFE programme for rehabilitating the withdrawn children from carpet weaving.

The major objectives of the present study are to:

- Estimate the magnitude of working children at the national level in general and in the hazardous occupations of carpet weaving in Mirzapur- Bhadhoi.
- Study the composition, characteristics, attendance and dropout rates of the enrolled children in these NFE schools, so as to find out, whether the basic objective of enrolling target children and imparting appropriate education has been achieved or not by these NFE schools.
- Evaluate the Non-formal education programme in terms of functions, amenities, teaching-learning materials, curriculum, and teachers training upgrades.
- Measure the level of skills learnt by the enrolled students

in these special schools/NFE schools. And also to measure the other achievements of the NFE schools in creating awareness among the people.

- Examine the impact and changes brought by the NFE programme, related to the elimination of child labour in the selected areas.
- Assess the community responses and acceptance of the NFE programme for imparting education and general awareness to the enrolled children.
- Prepare a set of recommendations for improving the quality of NFE programme so as to create positive impact and an appropriate response among the local community.

Methodology and Sample Survey

In order to achieve the above stated objectives, data was collected from field survey and secondary sources of information. The secondary sources of information include data collected from Ministry of labour, Government of India and Uttar Pradesh, NCERT, National and International voluntary organisations associated with rehabilitation of child labour in carpet weaving belt. The secondary data collected were analysed to identify the NFE schools in the belt. (Refer List of NFE schools, Annexure-I). Spatial distribution of these schools was worked out, so as to choose NFE centres from various spatial locations. The criteria adopted for the selection of NFE centres in the sample survey were:

- Rehabilitation agency and NGO concerned;
- Spatial location of the school;
- Year of establishment and multiplicity of activities undertaken in the schools.

Taking the above indicators into account, 58 NFE schools from various funding agencies, NGOs and spatial locations were selected. The field survey conducted covers 18 NGOs, 58 NFE centres, 311 children, 73 teachers and technical staff and 171 parents. The sample selected covers 22 blocks in 12 districts of Uttar Pradesh and Bihar. These 22 blocks represent carpet weaving core areas, peripheral zone and labour catchment zone. The sample survey coverage is given in Tables 1-3.

TABLE 1

Sample Survey Coverage

NGOs Surveyed	NFE Schools Surveyed	No. of Enrolled Children Surveyed		No. of Teacher Surveyed		No. of Parents of enrolled children Surveyed
		M	F	M	F	M
18	58	210	101	50	23	171

TABLE 2

Age and Sex Profile of Respondents

Respondent Groups	Sex Composition			%age Composition		
	T	M	F	Less than 20	20-40	Above 40
NGO Representatives	17	17	—	—	82	18
NFE School in-charge	58	42	16	19	78	3
Teachers	73	50	23	5	81	14
Parents of Enrolled Children	171	138	33	12	60	28

TABLE 3

Age and Sex Composition of Children Respondents

Respondent Children	Sex Composition			%age Composition			
	All	Boys	Girls	Less than 8	9-12	12-14	Above 14
Enrolled Children	311	210	101	11	78	9	2
Children Completed NFE	25	22	3	—	—	—	100

In addition to field observation and discussions held with NGO staff, teachers, children, parents of children and local community leaders, a structured questionnaire were prepared and filled by trained staff. 8 sets of questionnaires were prepared. The questionnaires prepared were for Rehabilitation agency, NGO staff, Child, teacher/staff of school, parent of child, child already completed NFE, loom owner and village community head. Questionnaire testing and pilot surveys were conducted in 4 NFE schools to examine the coverage and response of the respondents. Experts in consultation with respondents, monitored the field-testing at questionnaires, so as to prepare appropriate questions. Field testing and pilot survey was conducted for 15 days in Mirzapur, Sonabhadra, Saharsa and Bhadhoi. After an in-depth analysis of pilot survey in 4 NFE centers, final questionnaires were prepared.

The criteria adopted for the selection of respondents includes age, sex, caste and economic background of the family. The research team in the field selected the respondents after thorough discussions with NGOs and leaders of community members. Adequate measures were taken to create thorough understanding and rapport with the children and their families, so that correct data could be ascertained. The field staff stayed in the villages for 7 to 10 days initially, so as to familiarise with the local traditions, customs and manners. The survey commenced from 15th August and lasted till 15th November 1997.

Areal Extent of Carpet Weaving Belt in U.P. and Bihar

Hand knotted Carpet manufacturing in India is concentrated in Uttar Pradesh, Jammu and Kashmir and Rajasthan. The Mirzapur-Bhadohi belt in Uttar Pradesh holds the pre-eminent position in carpet weaving. According to AICMA survey in 1974,[17] out of total looms in Bhadohi-Mirzapur carpet belt, 62% looms were concentrated in Bhadohi, 18% in Mirzapur, 15% in Jaunpur and 4% in Allahabad district. The distribution of weavers recorded 62% in Bhadohi, 21% in Mirzapur, 12% in Jaunpur and 7% in Allahabad. These areas account for about 85-90%, of total value exported and 75% of total loomage in India.[18] The traditional carpet belt has far out-grown in terms of geographical spread. Both the growth in loomage and child weavers have been witnessed, in the area due to sudden demand of carpets for exports between 1985-1992.

Three carpet weaving zones have been identified taking into account, density of looms, nature of looms, type of labour and magnitude of child labour. The spatial expansion of areas covered by these three zones are presented in Table 4.

TABLE 4
Carpet weaving Zone and Labour Catchment Area—Areal Extent

Area/Zone	*District*	*Carpet Weaving Block/Areas*
Core Zone	1. Varanasi/ Bhadohi	(i) Bhadohi (ii) Gyanpur (iii) Sewapuri (iv) Araziline (v) Suriyawan (vi) Aurai (vii) Khamaria (viii) Maharajganj (ix) Ghosia (x) Gopiganj
	2. Mirzapur	(i) Kon (ii) City Block (iii) Lalganj (iv) Chunar
	3. Allahabad	(i) Handia (ii) Phulpur (iii) Pipari (iv) Saidabad (v) Phaphamau (vi) Hanumanganj
	4. Jaunpur	(i) Rampur (ii) Badshahpur (iii) Machhilishahr
Peripheral Zone	1. Mirzapur	(i) Hallia (ii) Marihan
	2. Son-Bhadra	(i) Dhorawal (ii) Dudhi
	3. Palamau	(i) Garhwa (ii) Lesliganj (iii) Daltanganj
	4. Banda	(i) Mau
	5. Allahabad	(i) Chail
	6. Jaunpur	(i) Kerakat
	7. Ghazipur	(i) Mohamadabad

Area/Zone	*District*	*Carpet Weaving Block/Areas*
Labour Catchment Zone	1. Saharsa (Bihar)	(i) Kosi Embankment Area
	2. Samastipur	(ii) Meheshi
	3. Patna	(i) Rosera (ii) Bihata (iii) Maner (iv) Bibhutipur
	4. Palamau	(i) Garhwa (ii) Daltenganj

Source: Field Work and Researchers Analysis done by research team.

The Core Zone

The core zone is the traditional carpet belt, a zone of 30 kms with heavy concentration of looms, operated by company branches as well as, by private loom holders. The core zone is characterised by intensive production. The incidence of hired and migrant child labour was found higher.[19] The 'core' carpet-weaving zone covers Bhadohi district and parts of Mirzapur, Allahabad and Jaunpur district.

The Peripheral Zone

The peripheral zone includes the district of Sonabhadra, Palamau, Ghazipur, Banda, Allahabad and Jaunpur. Carpet weaving in these areas were extended by implanting carpet looms in the newer areas through appointing agents, weaving contractors and loom holders. The contractors constructed looms in weaver's houses, by providing advance money to loom owners. The loom owner was obliged to take orders only from the contractor, irrespective of the wages offered. The main purpose was to avoid strict vigil imposed by Government and NGO's and to reach out for the cheap labour.[20] The expansion had been towards the South and Southeastern part, coinciding with the vast draught prone, flood prone, mono cropped and relatively backward Vindhyan-Kaimur plateau region. Most of the workers are either from family members of loom holders, or other workers from same village. Thus, this arrangement helps in transferring the onus of employing child labour to the families, to avoid legal prosecutions.

The Labour Catchment Zone

The area for drawing in child labour in the core and peripheral zone has expanded as far as Sharsa ,Purnea and Palamau districts in north east and south Bihar, Sidhi, Shahdol in Madhya Pradesh and Manipur-Karwi area of Banda (U.P.). The child labour is brought through well-organised network of labour procurers and suppliers by dubious means (false promises, inducements, and advance given to parents), pledging the children forever, against the advances and even kidnapping.

Carpet weaving Industry—Growth, Structure and Working Conditions

Carpet Weaving is an old craft industry in India. This craft was practiced as long back, as in 1300 B.C.[21] The painting of Ajanta and Elora also confirm that carpet-weaving industry was prevalent at that time. The king of Persia gifted a piece of carpet to the Mughal

Emperor, Akbar, the Great, in 16th century. Reference occur to the carpet making industry in northern India during the Mughal rule.[22] The artisans initially started carpet-weaving industry at Delhi, Lahore and Agra, but later it spread to other parts of India. Some artisans, on the way to Calcutta via G.T. Road, stayed at the village Modhosing and Ghosia, a place 20 kms away from Bhadohi. With the permission of king of Benaras, they started carpet weaving to earn their livelihood. These two villages have all along continued to enjoy reputation of excellence in carpet making. Gradually, the local people also learnt this art, which currently has spread to other districts and is now world famous as Mirzapur-Bhadhoi carpet belt.

Carpet Manufacturing—Export Value

At the time of independence, the value of carpets, exported from India stood at a mere Rs. 32 million (1947-48) and rose to Rs. 58 million during 1951-52 and was hovering around Rs. 55 million until 1960s. Nearly 90% of the Indian carpets were exported to European Countries and US during that period.[23]

In its foreign trade, the first major break came in 1970, when the value rose to Rs. 81 million. However, it is generally acknowledged even by official circles that this boost was mostly due to devaluation of Indian rupees (by a hefty 50%). Subsequently the exports rose to Rs. 360 million in 1974-75.

The major boost for the carpet industry was in 1985-86, due to the economic 'boom' in Iran, in the wake of rising oil prices. Consequently, the rising wage levels severely affected the production of carpets in Iran. The large displacement of child and women labour in carpet weaving in Iran, rose carpet prices sharply from Iran. Consequently, western importers turned to India, Pakistan, Nepal and China for the alternative source of supply. As a result the exports rose to Rs. 2450 million in 1985-86. Currently the exports in 1996-97 are around 580 million US $. The proportion of world carpet exports for India is around 17 to 20%, showing declining trends during last one decade, probably due to strict measures adopted by importers for humanizing the child labour and also proactive role adopted by major international NGOs to ensure consumer consensus. The other producers are Iran (26%), China (18%), Nepal (10%), Pakistan (8%) and Turkey (7%). Major importers of carpet from India are Germany (54%), USA (29%) and Other EEC Countries (14%).

TABLE 5

Carpet Exports From India 1947-97

Sr. No.	Year	Value (Millions)		% of World Total	Major Importers (as% of Total)		
		Indian Rupees	US $		USA	Germany	Other EEC
1.	1947-48	32					
2.	1951-52	58					
3.	1960-61	55					
4.	1965-66	37	7.8	5.8	33.1	6.3	57.3
4.	1970-71	81	10.9	5.7	44.4	21.1	33.2
5.	1975-76	359	41.5	7.9	26.2	51.0	14.6
6.	1980-81	1712	217.1	14.6	18.9	54.0	19.4
7.	1985-86	2447	336.9	21.6	32.7	46.3	14.7
8.	1990-91	5699	317.5	17.7	27.5	52.6	15.4
9.	1992-93	9167	347.1	17.9	28.8	53.7	13.9
10.	1996-97		580				

Source: The export figures significantly vary from source to source. The above table is worked out based on.

1. Census of India 1981, *Bhadhoi woolen carpet Industry.*
2. Juyal, B.N., *Child Labour in the Carpet Industry in Mirzapur Bhadhoi,* ILO, New Delhi.
3. Handicraft Department. Govt. of India.
4. GATT data bank.
5. CORT: Economics of Child Labour.

Carpet Industry Structure and Processes

The organization structure of the carpet industry is described as a simpler three-tier arrangement by the carpet businesses. These are:

- Manufacturer/Exporter
- Master Weaver and Loom Holder
- Weaver (Adults/Children). Both Family members and hired.

But in reality contractors constitute a separate category with a long line of "intermediaries" between the loom holder and the exporter/manufacturer. Another category of elite loom holders (non-artisans) has emerged as a separate category and a sizeable one in the recent times. Thus, the ownership of power has shifted from self-employed weavers to non-artisan dominant caste loom holder. In addition a series of middlemen are employed to help the manufacturer for completing the production demanded by the importers. Emergence of long line of intermediaries has siphoned away a major share of wages meant for weavers, leading to lower wages for the weavers. This is the major contributory factor to the exacerbation of the problem of child labour in carpet weaving.[24]

Carpet Manufacturing—Processes

Hand knotted carpet passes through various stages before final shape is given to it. Exporters receive woollen yarn from the agents/distributors of woolen mills. The woolen yarn is dyed in the dyeing factories. The dyeing of woolen yarn is now mostly done through chemicals as traditional natural vegetable colors used to fade away soon. Using of chemicals is harmful to children, as they inhale the fluff of woolen yarn. Designs, color combinations are prepared as per the orders from importers at the factory. The woolen yarn, cotton yarn, designs and color scheme are then distributed to loom holders through intermediaries. Monetary advance is paid to the loom holder towards the weaving charges.

At the loom holders place, winding of woolen yarn, stretching of warp and framing it to on looms are some of the major preliminary stages of weaving operation. These preparatory work is done by weaver with the help of children/women, and other adult weavers, before actual weaving operations commences. This preparatory works consume an average one week to 10 days. No remuneration is paid for the preparatory work.

Carpets are woven on vertical (upright) looms. The weft strings are tightly strung on the upper beam and the weaver separates alternate warp strings. In carpets of higher knottage, the weft strings are drawn very closely and the weaver has to pierce his fingers through them in order to draw the woolen thread. Depending upon the size, knottage, design and pile, completing a carpet can take one month to one year. The higher the quality, the more the labour input. There is an obvious relation with labour cost factor. Weaving and pre-final clipping at weavers level and beating of Knots are the main operation at the weaving stage in the households. Child Labour is used during preparatory work and weaving stage only

The woven carpet is sent to the factory for post weaving stages like; inspection, clipping, brushing, washing, drying, embossing and finishing. During the post weaving stages adult skilled labourers are employed. Thus the children's requirement for carpet manufacturing is at weaving stage, which is located in villages and not in the main factory. Hence Child Labour Act, 1986 is difficult to implement due to inaccessibility of looms located in far-flung villages. The Act specifies that, even if the child is found working in a premises of his/her family but if the employer for manufacturing purpose supplies the raw material, then the child work will be construed as work by the child in contravention of CLA Act, 1986 and the employer will be prosecuted as per the Supreme Court directions.

TABLE 6

Child Labour in Carpet Weaving

Age Group	*Preparatory work*			*Weaving*		*Post Weaving*
	Winding of Yarn	*Warp & weft. Framing colour Mixing*	*Dyeing of Yarn*	*Weaving*	*Clipping*	
8-10	98%	-		20%	-	-
11-12	100%	-		100%	20%	-
12-14	100%	-		100%	40%	-
15-20	-	80	-	100%	100%	100%
21 & Above	-	100	-	30	100%	100%

Source: Field Survey Conducted in the Study Area.

Carpet Weaving—Working Conditions

Several surveys conducted, shows that existing working conditions in the work places (looms) are highly unsuitable for long hours of arduous work of weaving especially for children. The plinth area is too small to provide comfortable sitting place to the weavers. Pits, where the weavers sit, does not have proper ventilation. Working space, seating capacity and lighting are insufficient in the weaving area. In addition the primitive technology, old and often dilapidated premises, improper and inadequate ventilation, over-crowding, air laden with wool fluff, haphazard and inconvenient layout are obvious limitations, under which weaving is carried out. More over there are no fixed hours of work. Working day usually consists of 8 to 10 hours.[25] If there is an urgent order to be delivered, the working hours are extended. Even if the workers are let-off late in the evening, they have to spend at least on hour on setting up things for the next morning e.g. wool sorting, ball making etc;

Magnitude of Child Labour in Carpet-Weaving Belt of Mirzapur-Bhadhoi

There have been numerous estimates of the number of workers and child labourers in the carpet industry. The estimates show a wide variation ranging from 100,000 to 500,000 child workers. Many of these estimates appear to have no factual basis and are suspected to be purposely exaggerated in order to make some preconceived point.[26]

As a part of government initiative in 1975, All India Carpet Manufacturers Association (AICMA) undertook a census of carpet looms in this region. This census simply counted the number of looms and weavers, size of looms operated and qualities woven. In the head count of weavers, there is no mention, whatsoever of child labour or child weaver. According to this census there were 26,731 looms and 73,420 weavers.[27] A 1985 survey found that out of 230,000 carpet workers in Mirzapur-Bhadhoi, the number of child workers was estimated to be around 75,000 (Kanbargi).[28] AICMA estimated 120,000 looms[29] in this region during 1986. A study done by Juyal estimated the number of child workers to be around 150,000 in 1987. Gupta confirms this figure of 150,000.[30]

A survey conducted by National Council of Applied Economic Research (NCAER) in 1992, placed the total child labour component in carpet weaving at approximately 8% of the total workforce, out of which 4.4% was family child labour. Hired child labour, including local as well as migratory child labour, was found to be 3.6%. Another survey conducted by NCAER in 1994 shows that there has been a decline in the percentage of hired child labour which has come down to 2.4%.[31]

Juyal estimated that carpet weavers in the region range between 500,000 and 750,000[32] in 1993. AICMA and other industry sources put it at about 500,000 carpet weavers (both adults and children). A study conducted by Juyal[33] in 5 selected rural/urban clusters, returned, 3456 adult and 7792 child workers in selected 2666 looms, depicting nearly 70% child labour component in the carpet weaving.

Carpet manufacturers point out the fault with these surveys. "The samples taken are microscopic as compared to total carpet industry and secondly most of these surveys were conducted in areas outside the main carpet weaving areas of the hub centre of the Bhadhoi-Mirzapur carpet belt, which is the north of the River Ganga, in the districts of Bhadhoi and surrounding it. The consequences have been that the samples taken for these surveys are not representative of the main carpet weaving area with the largest concentration of looms."[34]

TABLE 7

Child Labour Estimates—Mirzapur-Bhadhoi Carpet Weaving Belt

Name of Source	*Year*	*Numbers of Looms*	*Number of Weavers*	*Number of Child Weavers*	*% Child Weavers to total weavers*
AICMA	1975	26,731	73,420	N.A	N.A
Kanbargi	1985		230,000	75,000	33
AICMA	1986	120,000			
Juyal	1987			150,000	
Manju Gupta	1987			150,000	
NCAER	1992				8
Juyal	1993		650,000	450,000	70
CORT	1993		600,000**	120,000	22
Neera Burra	1995			1500,00	

** The survey assumed 600,000 weavers in the carpet weaving.

A study initiated by ILO and conducted by Centre for Operations Research and Training, Baroda in 1993 indicated 22% child weavers in the industry. The estimates worked were based on the sample study conducted in 362 carpet weaving enterprises covering 14 villages. The study assumed 6,50,000 weavers in the areas based on Juyal's estimates and concluded an estimated "1,20,000 child weavers and perhaps 1,30,000 children in the carpet industry" in Mirzapur-Bhadhoi belt.[35]

Neera Burra (1995) has estimated 1,50,000 child weavers in the Mirzapur- Bhadhoi carpet weaving belt.[36] This figure was quoted by the Hon'ble Supreme Court of India while delivering historic directions in 1996 for the eradication of Child Labour in India.

Estimated Out-of-School Children in Carpet Weaving Belt

An estimate of out-of-school children in the carpet-weaving belt of Mirzapur-Bhadhoi has been worked out considering projected population of children aged 5-14 years in 2001,based on the census projections. Percent of children attending schools in the age group of 5-14 years was assumed 61%, more than 5% points as stated in 1991 census for the carpet-weaving areas. The estimated out-of-school children are to the tune of 713,273 in the age group of 5-14 years. These children require immediate educational facilities.

Non-Formal Education Centers (NFE)—Spatial Distribution and Coverage

125 NFE special centers were located in the study area. 22 NFE special centers were in the Core zone, 73 in peripheral zone, and 29 in Catchment zone. Thus the distribution of NFE special centers is comparatively less than the requirement in the area, as the magnitude of villages without school facility is extremely high in the area. The location of the NFE schools is within the walking distance from the residence of enrolled children in the carpet belt. Majority of the schools are accessible by foot, even during the rainy season. The surroundings selected for the NFE schools are hygienically sound in Allahabad district, but incase of the other districts some of the schools are located in the congested areas where the approach is through unhygienic localities.

TABLE 8

Non-formal Education Special Centers Distribution (Block wise) 1997-98

Area	*Number of NFE Centers*
Core Area	22
Peripheral Area	73
Catchment Area	29
All Areas	124

The spatial distribution of NFE special centers depicts a highly concentrated pattern. Thus in order to bring other areas under the influence of the NFE special schools, NGOs should widen its base to new places. The site selection of NFE special centers should be in the areas, which are generally not severed by govt. schools and where the magnitude of child labour in carpet weaving is high. A pilot survey should be conducted in order to identify such areas, before locating a NFE special center.

The present survey found three instances where two or more than two NFE special centers are being operated in the same village by two different NGOs. The site selection of majority of NFE special centers is in accordance with objectives like, dominance of scheduled caste/schedule tribe and backward population areas, locations without government primary school and areas located in isolated and inaccessible belts.

NFE Special Centers—Children Enrollments

Among the 58 special NFE centers surveyed, 3259 children were enrolled in 1997 September. This works out to be 56 children per NFE centre. The proportion of girls in these NFE centres was 37%, which compared to all India level is significant. Most of the NGOs have been able to create conducive atmosphere in these rural areas for enrolling girls.

The age wise enrolment of children in the NFE special centers depicts, that 20% of the children were below 8 years of age, while 29% children were 8-10 years of age, 35% children were between 10-12 years, 12% children were between 12-14 years and the rest 4% were above 14 years of age. This indicates that a large proportion of children below 8 years also attended their NFE Centers. Thus, the objective of protecting younger children into weaving is being served. Children, who have devoted few years in carpet weaving, are reluctant to attend these NFE centers. However, it is encouraging to find that children between 8-12 years are encouraged for enrolment.

The social composition of children enrolled in the NFE Special Centers indicates, 44% of children were scheduled castes, 36% children were from other backward Classes (OBCs), 12% children were from Scheduled tribes and the rest 6% were from higher castes. Thus, the major objective of these centers has been to cover weaker sections of the Society, who are otherwise neglected in the education field. Majority of the NGOs have achieved the objective of covering weaker and marginal sections of the Society.

NFE Special Centers—Activities and Facilities

The NPE-1986 and NPCL-1987 envisaged Non-formal Education to provide basic primary education, vocational training, supplementary nutrition for children, stipend for children to compensate their earnings and health care for all the children attending these centers. The basic objective was to create general awareness for education and provide other child welfare programmes.

TABLE 9

NFE Schools—Age and Sex Enrollments

Enrollments in Special Schools			*% Girls Enrolled*	*Children Enrolled Per School*
Boys	*Girls*	*All*		
2040	1219	3259	37.40	56

Source: Based on Enrollment Registers of the Special Schools.

Majority of NFE special centers under study, in the Mirzapur-Bhadohi carpet-weaving belt, do not provide the above stated activities satisfactorily, due to paucity of funds. Even the NFE Programme provided by some centres is only for 2 or 3 years. Cooked midday meals are provided at few NFE centres. Provision of health care was extremely poor in majority of NFE centres except for Project Mala and Rugmark. They maintain regular health cards for the enrolled children and regular visits by doctors are ensured. Few NFE Centres also supply uniform and school bags.

NFE Special Centers—Infrastructure

If the NFE Special Centers are to attract and retain children, the infrastructure in terms of building, basic amenities, teaching aids, sports equipment and school environment must be provided satisfactorily. Due to initial heavy capital investment, majority of centers in India lack basic infrastructure facilities.

In a survey conducted by the Ministry of Education earlier, 40% centers have no pucca building, 9% have no building at all,

40% have no black-boards, 60% have no drinking water. 70% have no library facilities, 53% are without play grounds, 89% lack toilets and 35% have only a single teacher to teach three or four different classes. Many of these centers remain without any teacher for varrying periods of time. Even teachers are sub-contracted for teaching work.[37]

The study conducted for the NFE special centers in Mirzapur-Bhadohi belt, depicts the following results.

(i) 19% centres have pucca building, 10% centre semi-pucca and 71% centres have kutcha building. Only 12% buildings were self-owned and the rest were on rent. 15% centres had no building, the classes were held in open fields. During extreme heat, cold and rains no classes were held.

(ii) On an average each centre had 1.5 rooms. Two to three classes are taught simultaneously in each centre. Two classes are made to sit side by side and taught different courses. This diverts the attention of the students. Classes are generally held is the open fields, as rooms are congested and extremely small to accommodate all children. Ventilation is very poor in majority of centres and is not fit for teaching environment.

(iii) Only 32% centres have playgrounds and 52% centre have drinking water facility. Toilet facility was only available in few centres of Rugmark, and Project Mala.

The NFE special school infrastructure facilities are poor in majority of the centres. It is important that one time grant be given for the basic construction of infrastructure to the NGOs. In fact surroundings of the majority of centres are not conducive for NFE education. Stagnant water pools breeding mosquitoes were found in front of some NFE centres. Therefore adequate attention must be provided to site selection of NFE Centres. Local community/ Panchayats must be involved, so that proper building is earmarked for the NFE Centres.

NFE—Special Centres—Teaching Quality

Teachers are the key to education. They often represent the only positive role model, which children talk about and imbibe in the future. One pre-requisite of a successful education programme is the teaching methods and techniques adopted by teachers. The high drop-out/push-out rate is the outcome of improper teaching staff, who lack basic teaching skills. Therefore the appropriate choice of teacher's selection and regular in-service up-grade through training programmes is basic key to a successful NFE programme. The methods of teaching have to be joyful, demonstrative and participative. Rigid traditional teaching methods must give way to child—centred approaches.

Children must enjoy education, if it is to have a powerful effect. Unfortunately, most of the educational programmes suffer due to fewer attentions given for the recruitment of teachers. Wages given to teachers are exceptionally low. Many of them are forced to abandon teaching, or take second or even a third job in-order to survive. Teachers need to be retrained or replaced, if the education imparted is not relevant to children's needs. Teacher/children ratio also needs proper guidelines. High teacher/children ratio may not provide sufficient required guidance necessary for the children. The regular practice of teaching two different batches of students at the same time will also be counter productive for the education programme.

The 58 NFE special centers have recruited 151 staff (both teachers and supervisory staff) members. However majority of NFE centres had one or two staff members per centre. Total teaching staff excluding vocational teachers was 103 in these 58 NFE centres, registering an average of 1.77 teachers per centre.

Project Mala NFE centres take students regularly on year-to-year basis. All other NFE centres have only one batch of students in the entire two to three year periods. Sex ratio of teaching staff was 43 lady teachers per 100 male teachers. However few centres of Project Mala, have significant number of lady teachers. The teaching staff available and Teacher - Child ratio, reflects that several NFE centres need more recruitment of teachers. At least 2-teacher norm per NFE centre for every 50 children must be maintained in order to appropriately cater to the children's needs.

NFE—Special Centres—Teaching Staff Education Levels

The experience of several NFE centres throughout the country has shown that even less formal education level of the teachers with sufficient in-service training has helped to create proper education environment. It is difficult to find high formal educated teacher in these isolated and far flung areas, as the present wages paid to them are very low. Therefore teachers with appropriate formally-educated level, but trained properly are necessary for the successful NFE Programme.

62% teachers were educated up to 10+2 levels, 23% teachers up to graduation level and 15% above graduation level. Only 17% teachers were either experienced or trained, at the time of recruitment and 41% have joined at least one short-term teacher's training course. The distribution pattern of education levels and training attained by the teachers among the NFE centres, varied from NGO to NGO.

TABLE 10

Teachers Education Levels and Training

Total Teachers	*% Teachers Education Level*			*% Teachers*		*% Teachers attended short training*
	Up to 12	*Up to B.A.*	*Above B.A.*	*Trained*	*Untrained*	
103	62	23	15	17	83	41

The results of the study depicts, that training to recruited teachers must be given top priority, as still 60% teachers in NFE centres are without adequate training. Again the training courses should be organised by competent authority, which have wide-ranging experience. Staff from NCERT and State Training Institutes, should be engaged. The funding agencies should ensure proper in-service training of teachers and this condition should be made mandatory for the release of further funds. Several NFE centres, still follow old and traditional teaching methods that are boring and encourage drop out/push out rates. Training is one of the most important components envisaged in the NFE scheme. Paradoxically, the training component was lacking in the implementation process. It is rare to find teachers who have been specially trained for NFE programme. The question of less commitment, impulsiveness, hyperactivity, deficit attention disorders, poor speech pattern, inconsistency are familiar among the teachers, without basic training or in-service training. There are no easy remedies, though flexibility, creativity, humour, patience and a variety of curriculum based activity can help. Training is an essential ingredient to improve their ability.

NFE Special Centers—Curriculum Taught

The curriculum adopted and subjects taught in the NFE centres were diverse and ranging from basic skills of counting, alphabets learning, reading skills and numeric skills. Majority of NFE centres, followed self-devised curriculum by the teachers, and the teachers lacked experience for preparing the curriculum. The curriculum followed and subjects taught in majority of NFE centres lacked, proper guidance from NGOs and everything was left up to teacher's initiative. In the absence of trained teachers and lack of proper guidance, the effective NFE teaching programme is bound to suffer. This requires immediate attention from NGOs and funding agencies, as the purpose of NFE is self-defeating without appropriate curriculum followed. Although majority of the centres, do provide basic books, slates and stationery, but these items are provided only in the beginning of the term, and all such items are not provided subsequently. Children enrolled at later stages do not possess these items.

Most of the NFE special centers still follow the traditional and unimaginative methods of education, relay on outdated teaching methods without concentrating on practical demonstrations, out door visits, usage of charts, flash cards, posters and other co curricular activities. However, NFE centers using these teaching aids have shown positive impact on the educational understanding of the children. Teachers with in-service training courses were trying to adopt the new techniques. Students were found attentive and engrossed in the classes, where practical demonstration of skill was shown are used.

NFE Special Centres—Skill Test Performance

In an earlier study conducted by the NCERT during 1992-93 in 46 low literacy districts across eight states, the result of skills learnt by children were tested. The study indicated;[38]

(i) Among class V students, the maximum student achievement was 20 out of 40 in word meaning and 17 out of 44 in reading comprehension.

(ii) Learning achievements in mathematics were even lower than in reading. More than four-fifth of the students studying in class IV or V could not achieve a minimum score of 40 per cent.

Jacob Aikara, conducted a study in the year 1997, in four states to assess the level of learning achievements in Language, Mathematics and Environmental Studies.[39] The study observed that the students performed better in language as compared to the other two subjects. The study also showed that there was marginal difference in the performance of boys and girls in Language and Environmental Studies. But in Mathematics boys had significantly higher score than girls.[40]

In the case of present study, teachers were asked about the examination method followed in the NFE schools for testing the skills of the enrolled children. In majority of cases no examination was conducted systematically. However, in case of few NFE schools monthly progress of the children was recorded. In order to examine and assess the skills achieved by children in the selected NFE schools, a skill test was conducted, covering skills related to understanding Arithmetic, language reading and language writing, General Awareness, Civic Sense, Environmental Science, History and Geography of local area. Simple age appropriate and learner specific questions on the above aspects were prepared, keeping in view the local and community understanding. The selected children were asked to write the answers on separate sheets. Reading tests along with verbal question-answer were also conducted. The results of the tests conducted by the research team depict the following:

(i) Only 11% children have good level of understanding, 39% were average and the rest 49% were poor

(ii) Arithmetic skills were good only for 13% children, where as it was poor for 34% and moderate for 53%.

(iii) General knowledge skills were poor for 60% children and average for 34%.

(iv) Civic sense skills were comparatively better, probably due to regular infusion of these values by teachers.

(v) Environmental Science skills were found extremely poor for 83% children, where as 15% were found moderate in these skills.

(vi) The knowledge of local history and geography were also

found below the mark for majority of the children.

(vii) The reading and writing skills were found better among majority of children.

The performance of boys and girls did not show significant variations. In fact, girls scored better in terms of reading, writing and environmental science. Boys performed better in arithmetic and general understanding. Performance of other skills was similar between boys and girls. The results of the test varied among the NFE centres depending upon the motivating and training level of the teachers.

The skill test performance of the selected children was highly correlated with education level of teachers and teaching training level. This proves that educational understanding levels of children are closely associated with teachers quality, methods of teaching employed by teacher, school environment in terms of infrastructure and facilities provided in these centres.

TABLE 11

Skill Test Results
Per cent Children Tested

Skill learnt & level of understanding			*Arithmetic Skill*			*General Knowledge*			***Civic Sense Skill***		
Good	*OK*	*Poor*	*Good*	*OK*	*Poor*	*Good*	*OK*	*Poor*	*Good*	*OK*	*Poor*
11.8	39.1	49.1	13.4	52.9	33.7	5.8	33.8	60.4	24.0	23.6	52.4

The responses from the parents were encouraging as 70 per cent parents were taking keen interest about child's education by attending parent-teacher meetings. 87% parents were sending children regularly to schools, however discussion with some parents indicated that absenteeism among girls was more due to the requirement of girls for domestic work during peak season when employment is in demand, while others felt that they needed separate schools for girls. Some parents also wanted lady teachers should teach girl students in the formal schools. The results of the survey point out that 74% parents wanted to pursue formal education for the children after completing the NFE course. 21% felt children are required to work along with the families after the NFE course, while 5% respondents had no idea and indicated wait and watch attitude. When the same questions were asked to the enrolled children, the answers matched with that of the parents. 75% children wanted to attend formal schools, while 13% wanted to enter into labour market and 12% were without any clue or idea about their future.

Parents were asked to rank the changes noticed in the child after attending the NFE classes. Response from parent indicated that positive changes were found in case of behavior, general awareness and cleanliness and hygiene. However 8% respondents felt that respect and attitude towards parents and elders was diminishing. Parents also thought that in few cases (15%) children were reluctant to help in family work.

Recommendations

- NGOs must conduct prior survey and identify only out-of-school children for enrolments in these schools.
- Areas to be selected for NFE schools should be carefully chosen especially those areas, where primary school facility is not available.
- Orientation course for NGOs should be given to familiarise the Non-formal Education requirements.
- Preference for enrollments in these schools should be given to older out-of-school children, while younger children should be enrolled in formal schools.
- Vocational Training for the enrolled children should be identified taking into account the resource base and market demand of the area.
- Stipend of Rs. 100 should be given only to children withdrawn from work and not all children. Instead the money should be utilized for providing books, uniforms, school bags, recruitment of more teachers and enrollment of more children.
- Development of basic infrastructure in schools likes; mats, drinking water, toilets should be provided.
- In-service training programme for all recruited teachers should be made compulsory for at least once in a year.
- NFE system to be integrated with state education system,

to smoothen transition of children from NFE to formal education system.

- Acceleration of co-ordination among various departments to converge all activities in the areas.
- Networking of NGOs should be strengthened and encouraged for sharing experiences.
- The NFE curriculum should be standardized and a committee of experts should identify textbooks.
- Regular Institutional assessment of the NFE programme should be conducted by the funding agencies.
- One time grant for maintenance of infrastructure, purchase of teaching kits, books for the library, vocational training equipments and raw materials for training should be made available to the NGOs.

References

1. The Government of India acceded to this convention on 11th December 1992. The convention of the Rights of the child enshrines as interdependent and indivisible the full range of the civil, political, economic, social and cultural rights of all children that are vital to their survival, development, protection and participation in the lives of their societies. One of the tenets of the convention is that all actions concurring children, their best interests should be taken fully into account. Article 32 *recognizes* children's right to be protected from work that threatens their health, education or development and enjoins states, to set minimum ages for employment and to regulate working conditions.
2. ILO Report, (1995), *Child Labour, Targeting the intolerable.*
3. As of December 2000, the Bill had yet to find its way into the Statute book. But the mere threat of such a measure panicked the general industry of Bangladesh. Child workers, mostly of them girls were summarily dismissed from the garment factories and India was pressurized to implement strictly the Child Labour Act, 1986.
4. Sheridan Bartlett (1999): *Cities for Children, Children's Rights, Poverty and Urban Management,* UNICEF, Earthscan Publication Limited, London, pp. 216-217
5. Weiner, Myron (1990): *The Child and the state in India,* Oxford University Press, New Delhi,
6. *Ibid.*
7. The PROBE Team (1999): Public Report on Basic Education in India, Oxford University Press, New Delhi, p. 1.
8. The PROBE Team (1999): Public Report on Basic Education in India, Oxford University Press, New Delhi, pp. 17.
9. *Ibid.*

10. *Op. cit.*, 29.
11. Weiner, Myron (1991): *The Children and the State in India*, Oxford University Press, New Delhi.
12. This has been one of the strategy adopted in Kerela and Himachal Pradesh, where very low school dropout rates are matched by low incidence of child labour.
13. National Education Policy (1986): *A programme of Action*, New Delhi, Government of India.
14. Anil Bordia (1977): *Working paper on Child Labour in India*, Working paper on child labour in India, pp. 11-12 and 99, Ministry of Education and Social Welfare.
15. Ministry of Labour (1998), *Policy and Programme for the Rehabilitation of Working Children and Manual for the Implementation of National Child Labour Projects*.
16. Ministry of Labour document giving list of Existing National Child Labour Projects as on 06-06-2000. Figures in brackets indicate number of district covered under the programme.
17. A ICMA (1974): *Census of Hand knotted Carpets, Mirzapur*.
18. Juyal, B.N. (1993): *Child Labour is the Carpet Industry in Mirzapur-Bhadohi*, ILO. New Delhi.
19. Juyal, B.N., *Ibid*.
20. Juyal, B.N., *Ibid*.
21. Agarwal, G.N., 1979: *Carpet-e-world*, Vol. 1, p. 100.
22. Abul-Fazal, *Aine-I-Akbari*.
23. Juyal, B.N. (1993): *Child Labour in the carpet industry in Mirzapur-Bhadohi: A situational analysis and evaluation of government of India's National Child Labour Project*, ILO, New Delhi.
24 *Op. cit.*, No. 14.
25. Katagade, 1984
26. Richard Anker, Sandhya Barge, Shahid Ashraf and Deborah Levison (1998): "Economics of Child Labour in India's Carpet Industry", in *Economics of Child Labour in Hazardous Industries, Edited*, CORT, Baroda.
27. Census of India, 1981: *Bhadhoi Woollen Carpet Industry*, UP, Part -XC, Series - 22.
28. Kanbargi , R. (1988): *op. cit.*
29. Juyal, B.N. (1993): *Child Labour in the carpet industry in Mirzapur-Bhadhoi: A situational analysis and evaluation of government of India's National Child Labour Project*, ILO , New Delhi.
30. Gupta, M. (1989): *Child Labour in hazardous work in India; Situation and Policy Experience* unpublished study of ILO.
31. NCAER (1994): "Child Labour in Carpet Industry," Margin, October-December 1994.
32. Juyal. B.N. (1993): *op. cit.*
33. Juyal, B.N. (1993): *op. cit.*
34. Sharma, V.R. (1998): "Economics of Child Labour in Carpet Industry", In *Economics of Child Labour in Hazardous Industries, Edited*, CORT, Baroda.
35. Richard Anker, Sandhya Barge, Shahid Ashraf and Deborah Levison

(1998) : " Economics of Child Labour in India's Carpet Industry", in *Economics of Child Labour in Hazardous Industries*, Edited, CORT, Baroda.

36. Burra, N. (1995): Born to work: Child Labour in India, Oxford University Press, New Delhi.
37. Ministry of Education Report, p. 36.
38. UNICEF (1996): *Progress of the States.*
39. Yadav, M.S and Others (2000), EDUCATION FOR ALL, Learner Achievement in Primary Schools, MHRD, GOI and NIEPA.
40. *Ibid.*

ANNEXURE 1

Carpet Weaving and Catchment Belt Local NGOs and Non-formal Education Schools

Sr. No.	NGO Name	Districts Covered	Name of NFE Schools	Name of NFE Schools Selected for Survey
1.	Swami Vivekanand Siksha Samiti (SVSS)	Mirzapur	1. Mujhera Khurd 2. Mujhera Kalan 3. Bhogan 4. Mavai Kalan 5. Bahuti	1. Mujhera Khurd 2. Mujhera Kalan 3. Bhogan 4. Bahuti
2.	Bachapan Bachao Andolan (BBA)	Mirzapur Sonbhadra	1. Purikatra 2. Ghabi Ghat 3. Jorukhad 4. Parsi Tola 5. Hinshinpur	1. Purikatra 2. Jorukhad
3.	Manav Sansadan Mahila Vikas Sansthan (MS&MVS)	Bhadohi	1. Amva 2. Paniyara 3. Jegapur	1. Amva 2. Paniyara
4.	Yuva Vikas Sansthan (YVS)	Ghazipur	1. Salempur 2. Narayanpur	1. Salempur 2. Narayanpur
5.	Gramodaya Sansthan (GS)	Banda	1. Balapur 2. Matiyara 3. Media ka Dera 4. Biki ka Dera 5. Bhatla	1. Balapur 2. Matiyara 3. Media ka Dera
6.	Ankur Foundation (AF)	Sonbhadra	1. Biluroa 2. Dhanavathan 3. Longa 4. Mithunia 5. Singha 6. Asan Bandh 7. Goura Singha 8. Barvahi Kholi 9. Jharia 10. Neemiyachee 11. Ghidia 12. Kaillul 13. Khempur 14. Chekhwaheed 15. Kon 16. Ramgarh 17. Kachnarwa	1. Biluroa 2. Dhanavathan 3. Longa 4. Mithunia 5. Neemiyachee 6. Ghidia 7. Gorasigha 8. Chekhwaheed 9. Kon 10. Ramgarh

(Contd.)

Sr. No.	NGO Name	Districts Covered	Name of NFE Schools	Name of NFE Schools Selected for Survey
7.	Arpan Gramin Vikas (AGV)	Patna	1. Bahpur 2. Patsi 3. Sikandarpur 4. Maner 5. Pandechak 6. Bahusi 7. Lodipur 8. Baank 9. Manergarh 10. Bihata 11. Bajitpur 12. Dyalchak	1. Bahpur 2. Maner 3. Baank 4. Manergarh 5. Bihata 6. Bajitpur
8.	Kosi Sewa Sadan (KSS)	Saharsa	1. Kothia 2. Arapatti 3. Jhutiki 4. Moyalasthan 5. Mahishi	1. Jhutiki 2. Koyalasthan 3. Mahishi
9.	Sampurna Gramin Vikas Kendra (SGVK)	Palamau	1. Chakka 2. Kala Phar 3. Kurin Patro 4. Duela	1. Chakka 2. Kala Pahar 3. Kurin Patro
10.	SAMUDAYA	Samastipur Begusarai	1. Muradpur 2. Mathudumar 3. Modipur 4. Kander 5. Udaipur 6. Govindpur 7. Shankarbarsa 8. Rajwara 9. Milky 10. Samastipur city 11. Koksha 12. Sihama	1. Muradpur 2. Kanker 3. Shankarbarsa 4. Rajwara 5. Milky 6. Koksha 7. Sihama
11.	SACCS/BBA	New Delhi	1. Mukti Ashram Mohammadpur	1. Mukti Ashram
12.	Project Mala (PM)	Mirzapur	1. Guria 2. Hasra 3. Amoi 4. Pathera	1. Guria 2. Hasra

(Contd.)

Sr. No.	*NGO Name*	*Districts Covered*	*Name of NFE Schools*	*Name of NFE Schools Selected for Survey*
13.	CREDA*	Mirzapur Bhadohi Sonbhadra	1. Bikna 2. Lakhnia 3. Kaval 4. Dhuma	1. Bikna 2. Lakhnia 3. Kaval 4. Dhuma
14.	RUGMARK Foundation	Bhadohi	1. Gopiganj	1. Gopiganj
15.	Bandhu Mukti (Manch (BMM)	Sonbhadra	1. Jorukhurd 2. Mithunia	1. Jorukhurd
16.	Child Eradication and welfare Society (CLE & WS)	Bhadohi	1. Newada Kalan	1. Newada Kalan
17.	Child Welfare Society (CWS)	Mirzapur Bhadohi	1. Lalli 2. Parsona 3. Karsouta 4. Phoolwari 5. Browdhi 6. Sirsace 7. Majuhari 8. Noogdova 9. Madhka 10. Parsiya 11. Imliphokhar	1. Lalli 2. Parsona 3. Karsauta
18.	Samangra Gramin Vikas Sansthan (SGVS)	Sonbhadra	1. Jorukhad 2. Gheevki 3. Keval 4. Dhuma 5. Madni Khurd	1. Jorukhad 2. Gheevki 3. Keval

*Other NFE centres of CREDA were stopped temporarily due to stoppage of funds from Ministry of Labour (India). Data from CREDA was not available.

TABLE 1

Carpet Weaving and Catchment Belt Local NGOs and Non-formal Education Schools

Sr. No.	*NGO Name*	*Districts Covered*	*Name of NFE Schools*	*Name of NFE Schools Selected for Survey*
1.	Swami Vivekanand Siksha Samiti (SVSS)	Mirzapur	6. Mujhera Khurd 7. Mujhera Kalan 8. Bhogan 9. Mavai Kalan 10. Bahuti	5. Mujhera Khurd 6. Mujhera Kalan 7. Bhogan 8. Bahuti
2.	Bachapan Bachao Andolan (BBA)	Mirzapur Sonbhadra	6. Purikatra 7. Ghabi Ghat 8. Jorukhad 9. Parsi Tola 10. Hinshinpur	1. Purikatra 2. Jorukhad
3.	Manav Sansadan Mahila Vikas Sansthan (MS&MVS)	Bhadohi	4. Amva 5. Paniyara 6. Jegapur	3. Amva 4. Paniyara
4	Yuva Vikas Sansthan (YVS)	Ghazipur	3. Salempur 4. Narayanpur	3. Salempur 4. Narayanpur
5.	Gramodaya Sansthan (GS)	Banda	6. Balapur 7. Matiyara 8. Media ka Dera 9. Biki ka Dera 10. Bhatla	4. Balapur 5. Matiyara 6. Media ka Dera
6.	Ankur Foundation (AF)	Sonbhadra	18. Biluroa 19. Dhanavathan 20. Longa 21. Mithunia 22. Singha 23. Asan Bandh 24. Goura Singha 25. Barvahi Kholi 26. Jharia 27. Neemiyachee 28. Ghidia 29. Kaillul 30. Khempur 31. Chekhwaheed 32. Kon 33. Ramgarh 34. Kachnarwa	11. Biluroa 12. Dhanavathan 13. Longa 14. Mithunia 15. Neemiyachee 16. Ghidia 17. Gorasigha 18. Chekhwaheed 19. Kon 20. Ramgarh

(*Contd.*)

Sr. No.	NGO Name	Districts Covered	Name of NFE Schools	Name of NFE Schools Selected for Survey
7.	Arpan Gramin Vikas (AGV)	Patna	13. Bahpur 14. Patsi 15. Sikandarpur 16. Maner 17. Pandechak 18. Bahusi 19. Lodipur 20. Baank 21. Manergarh 22. Bihata 23. Bajitpur 24. Dyalchak	7. Bahpur 8. Maner 9. Baank 10. Manergarh 11. Bihata 12. Bajitpur
8.	Kosi Sewa Sadan (KSS)	Saharsa	6. Kothia 7. Arapatti 8. Jhutiki 9. Moyalasthan 10. Mahishi	4. Jhutiki 5. Koyalasthan 6. Mahishi
9.	Sampurna Gramin Vikas Kendra (SGVK)	Palamau	5. Chakka 6. Kala Phar 7. Kurin Patro 8. Duela	4. Chakka 5. Kala Pahar 6. Kurin Patro
10.	SAMUDAYA	Samastipur Begusarai	13. Muradpur 14. Mathudumar 15. Modipur 16. Kander 17. Udaipur 18. Govindpur 19. Shankarbarsa 20. Rajwara 21. Milky 22. Samastipur city 23. Koksha 24. Sihama	8. Muradpur 9. Kanker 10. Shankarbarsa 11. Rajwara 12. Milky 13. Koksha 14. Sihama
11.	SACCS/BBA	New Delhi	2. Mukti Ashram Mohammadpur	1. Mukti Ashram
12.	Project Mala (PM)	Mirzapur	5. Guria 6. Hasra 7. Amoi 8. Pathera	3. Guria 4. Hasra

(*Contd.*)

Sr. No.	NGO Name	Districts Covered	Name of NFE Schools	Name of NFE Schools Selected for Survey
13.	CREDA*	Mirzapur Bhadohi Sonbhadra	5. Bikna 6. Lakhnia 7. Kaval 8. Dhuma	5. Bikna 6. Lakhnia 7. Kaval 8. Dhuma
14.	RUGMARK Foundation	Bhadohi	1. Gopiganj	1. Gopiganj
15.	Bandhu Mukti (Manch (BMM)	Sonbhadra	3. Jorukhurd 4. Mithunia	1. Jorukhurd
16.	Child Eradication and welfare Society (CLE & WS)	Bhadohi	1. Newada Kalan	1. Newada Kalan
17.	Child Welfare Society (CWS)	Mirzapur Bhadohi	12. Lalli 13. Parsona 14. Karsouta 15. Phoolwari 16. Browdhi 17. Sirsace 18. Majuhari 19. Noogdova 20. Madhka 21. Parsiya 22. Imliphokhar	4. Lalli 5. Parsona 6. Karsauta
18.	Samangra Gramin Vikas Sansthan (SGVS)	Sonbhadra	6. Jorukhad 7. Gheevki 8. Keval 9. Dhuma 10. Madni Khurd	4. Jorukhad 5. Gheevki 6. Keval

*Other NFE centres of CREDA were stopped temporarily due to stoppage of funds from Ministry of Labour (India). Data from CREDA was not available.

APPENDIX

Recommendations for Rehabilitation of Released Children from Work

Recommendations:

The recommendations derived were related to:

1. Generation of employment opportunities.
2. Co-ordination to integrate government efforts, with voluntary organizations for the effective utilization of poverty alleviation programmes and general development programmes.
3. Strengthening, monitoring and evaluation of NFE special schools.
4. Awareness generation programmes.

I. Generation of employment Programmes

- The incomes decreased due to the withdrawal of children from looms, has also closed a source of taking loans/ advances. Thus job opportunities for adults must be created. There are sizeable number of grown up children and parents having adequate knowledge of the art of carpet weaving. Number of families also possesses looms, but they don't have requisite knowledge of acquiring credit facilities and marketing expertise. ***Promotion of Co-operatives for carpet manufacturing would ensure full employment and higher adult wages.***
- Training and financial aid for parents of enrolled children in industrial crafts like; sewing and dress making, candle making, machine weaving, tufted carpet weaving, food

processing, agro- based activities like; dairy farming and goatry should be started in the NFE centres. The training and financial aid should be arranged through government sponsored poverty alleviation programmes. The emphasis should be on self-employment, income supplementation through development plans for informal sector as a part of anti-poverty strategy.

- Parents of enrolled children should get priority under various poverty alleviation programmes of government. These programmes include, Employment Assurance Scheme (EAS), Integrated Rural Development Programme (IRDP), Jawahar Rozgar Yojana (JRY), Development of Women and Children in Rural Areas (DWCRA), District Primary Education Programme (DPEP), Integrated Child Development Services (ICDS), National Literacy Campaigns (NLCs), School Health Projects (SHP), Training for Rural Youth for self employment (TRYSEM), Indira Awas Yojana (IAY), Prime Minister's Rozgar Yojana (PMRY), Mid-day meal scheme, etc.; NGO's must help the parents to get loans and other entitlements under these programmes. This would help in bringing confidence building measures with the community.

II. Co-ordination Committee

- Co-ordination between government agencies, representatives of NGO's and parents of enrolled children in the NFE special schools is basic pre-requisite condition to successful implementation of government programmes. ***District level committees for convergence of services should be set up for this purpose.***
- The Committee should be headed by district collector, other members should include representatives of related government departments associated with above stated poverty alleviation programmes, representatives of NGO's associated with child labour eradication programmes and Non-formal education programmes, representatives of parents of enrolled children in NFE schools and representatives of village Panchayats. The representatives of village panchayats should include

weaker sections and women.

- The Committee should accord priorities to the affected families under the above stated, poverty alleviation programmes.

III. Strengthening, Monitoring and Evaluation of NFE Programme

- The magnitude of villages without, schooling facility is high in the carpet-weaving belt. Instead of opening new government schools (which are currently in-effective and incapable of imparting relevant education for the rural needs), more Non-Formal Education schools must be opened by providing funds to the NGO's with proven record of NFE. It would ensure proper educational environment in the carpet weaving belt and would stop entry of younger children into weaving as well as provide required education to the children withdrawn from carpet weaving.
- The location of NFE schools should proceed with proper survey for the identification of areas. Areas with high incidence of child labour in carpet weaving must be selected for NFE school location. The site location of the school should consider the accessibility of villages to be covered for NFE programme. Location of the NFE School should be central, so that majority of children from surrounding villages could get enrolled in the schools. Other considerations for site location should include areas dominant with scheduled caste/ other backward castes/economically weaker sections and scheduled tribe population. Funding agencies should ensure that sites selected are hygienically sound and appropriate. NGO's should also approach village panchayats for providing building facility for the school. Separate classrooms/sitting place for teaching different level of classes must be provided.
- To wean away children from work and motivate them to join NFE program, camp schools should be organised for four to eight weeks in the block/tehsil headquarters in a pleasant or child friendly environment, before the

academic session. Social workers/teachers should visit regularly to the children in work place and develop positive relationship with parents before motivating them to send children for such camps. The motivation requires highly oriented, talented and trained staff. These camps should remain full time and should provide books, stationery, shelter and food.

- Non-Formal Education strategy in the present form will prove in-effective, unless children completed NFE are not enrolled in formal schools or are not provided apprenticeship training to avail self employment. Thus children should be either enrolled in formal schools or be retained by these NFE schools till 15 years of age. The Two/Three years of NFE programme may not be suitable for a child who has entered in the schools at the age of 7/8 years.
- Preference in enrolments in these NFE schools should be given to working children from scheduled castes/ scheduled tribes/other backward classes and economically weaker sections. However other children or siblings of these children should also be encouraged to get enrolled in formal schools or in these NFE schools. Adequate steps must be taken to enrol girl children in these NFE schools.
- NFE schools must provide multiplicity of functions viz.; Non-formal education, nutritional diet, medical care, supply of books, stationery (slates, chalks, notebooks etc.;). At least one vocational training course should be included along with NFE. The vocational course should be area specific, depending upon local crafts, resources and demand. After the completion of three years of NFE, relevant apprenticeship training and trade training information must be given to the children not enrolled in formal schools. (including information regarding credit facilities available and further training programmes conducted by government.)
- NFE school timings and vocation period should be fixed in consultation with community members. It should be conducive to the agricultural calendar of the area.
- The teachers of NFE School must undertake adult

education programme once in a week for the parents of enrolled children at the time suitable to them. It will create child/ teacher/parent rapport, improve children attendance and will discourage dropout rates.

- The stipend for the enrolled children should be restricted to one child per family, while other children from the same family should be encouraged to join schools. The stipend should be converted into a rehabilitation fund to be given only after the completion of NFE programme. The rehabilitation fund must be regularly deposited in bank/post office against the child's name. The rehabilitation fund could be used either for further schooling or for the purchase of equipment's for self-employment. The stipend value may vary from NGO to NGO, depending upon funds available for the purpose.
- Transitory rehabilitation centres must be opened in the carpet weaving belt for the released children from bondage on the same pattern as is done in Mukti Ashram in New Delhi (SACCS/BBA). The maintenance and operational funds for this purpose should be collected from the employer's (Supreme Court directions must be followed to collect funds). The transitory camp should provide basic NFE and vocational skills for 6 to 12 months.
- A minimum norm of two teachers per NFE school for 50 children must be implemented. Teachers recruited for the NFE program holds the key for the success of programme. To procure talented teachers, salaries of teachers must be increased to minimum of Rs. 1500 per month. Committed teachers (both males and females) preferably from local areas and from dominant social groups, even with less formal education level should be recruited. NGO's must ensure that all recruited teachers are provided teaching training programme at the beginning of the session. Regular in-services training up-grades, should be conducted by experts from NCERT/ State Educational Training Institutes. The training up-grades should be at least once in a year.
- The aim of the in-service training is to enhance the quality of the work of teachers/supervisors. The training should

be based on "activity based instructions" like; providing learning activities, promoting learning by doing, using local environment, creating an interesting class room, preparation of lesson plans, improvisation of teaching aids.

- The teachers should be given coloured paper, gum, scissors, drawing pins, cardboard, geometrical instruments, in the form of a kit. Each school should sanction Rs.500 per annum towards supply of teaching material kit. The teachers should also be supplied with teachers handbooks with instructions in mathematics, environmental studies, containing lesson plans, which is prepared by practising teachers and experts.
- Regular visits to surrounding areas for children enrolled especially to post office, health centre and neighbouring fields, must be encouraged, so that the children become more aware of the environment and community. At times community leaders, policy makers like police officers, doctors etc.; should be called at the NFE centres, to have free exchange of views with children.
- Teachers of several NFE centres should meet once in a month, to exchange their experiences. The participation in these meetings will enrich their knowledge in the process of instruction. It helps them to know about different types of individuals and group activities. They can get their doubts cleared with the help of teachers educators.
- NGO's should ensure that teachers employ joyful, demonstrative and participative methods to inculcate educational skills to the enrolled children. Rigid and traditional teaching methods must give way to child centred approaches of teaching. The teaching methods should include, our-door environmental trips, demonstrative experiments, cultural programmes, sport activities, songs, drama, paining competitions and testing of skills learn by the children.
- The curriculum adopted and subjects to be taught in the NFE schools must follow either State Board Primary Education levels or Minimum Levels of Learning prepared by NCERT. NGO's must monitor and supply

monthly targets of curriculum to be completed by teachers. State Education Boards should ease procedures for conducting examination to the children from these NFE schools. A set of modal question papers should be circulated by NGO's to the teachers, so those students are well prepared to face the examinations.

- NGO's teachers and other workers must evolve efforts to inculcate general awareness related to moral values, public health, preservation of natural environment, cleanliness, civic and sentry sense among the children. Presentation of awards for best groups of children projecting and implementing these skills should be promoted.
- Data regarding children enrolled their age, sex, caste, previous work occupation, their attendance rate, dropout rates must be regularly maintained by NFE staff. The information should be supplied to the funding agencies as and when required.
- Funding agencies should conduct regular performance assessment of NFE programme. The assessment committee should be independent not associated with funding agency or NGO. The body should have powers to inspect special schools and take follow-up action. The body should assess the competencies of children enrolled in special schools and also evolve a mechanism to deal with children coming out of such schools for further studies. The mechanism evolved should provide education in primary and secondary schools for further education or provide necessary apprenticeship training. The body should suggest methods to deal with special schools not functioning properly. The release of funds should be automatic on receipt of report from the assessment committee.
- Release of funds should be regular, so that NFE program is not stopped in between. The stoppage of NFE program by NGOs in between gives wrong signals to the society and can effect the whole NFE program. If NGOs are found effective in inparting NFE by funding agencies, alternate arrangements must be made without stopping the already existing schools.

- The budget estimates stipulated under various heads should include One time special grant for building infrastructure, purchase of teaching aids and materials, books for library, sports equipment's, vocational training equipment's and other necessary infrastructure. The grant released must be utilised for the specified purpose only. Per child per annum expenditure should be raised to Rs. 3000 minimum.
- Special preference for opening NFE schools in the Peripheral zone and Child Labour Catchment zone should be given.

Sanction of funding for opening of NFE schools by local NGO's should be guided by Performance of NGO in creating mass awareness and propagating eradication of child labour in carpet weaving.

- Community rapport created by NGO in the area.
- Survey and identification of children (details about family's social, economic position) to be covered by NFE program.
- Site selection with identification of building to be used for NFE programme (The building could be either rented/provided by local community or to be constructed).
- Before final recommendation for sanction of NFE School, a team should visit the site and talk to community leaders. Once satisfied the project should be recommended for financial support.

Awareness Generation

The awareness generation strategy should aim at:

- Mobilizing public opinion for creating community participation for educational environment for children and elimination of full time child labour.
- Sensitizing all section of society, particularly the literate society.
- Formation of people's committee's at various levels.
- Involve various social, political and cultural movements.

The objectives would be achieved by—

- Launching a publicity blitz, through electronic and print media, to sensitise society against child labour. Modes of awareness could be posters, stickers, slogans including songs, newspapers, bulletin, calendars, wall hangings, hoarding, banners, wall writing, regular advertisements, cultural shows, rallies, music padyatras, street corner meetings, formation of human chain, folk songs and dramas, debates, essay competition, quiz competition etc.
- To create awareness among parents and children at work about deleterious effect of sending children to work and significance of education.
- Morality, social and legal consciousness should be generated against employers.

Index